Contents

Graham R Foster PhD FRCP
Reader in Hepatology
Imperial College Faculty of Medicine
Lead Clinician
Liver Unit
St Mary's Hospital
London

Robert D Goldin MD FRCPath
Senior Lecturer in Histopathology
Imperial College Faculty of Medicine
Consultant Histopathologist
Department of Histopathology
St Mary's Hospital
London

MARTIN DUNITZ

© 2002 Martin Dunitz Ltd, a member of the Taylor & Francis Group

First published in the United Kingdom in 2002
by Martin Dunitz, an imprint of Taylor and Francis Group, 11 New Fetter Lane, London EC4P 4EE

Reprinted in 2002

Tel.:   +44 (0) 20 7583 9855
Fax: +44 (0) 20 7842 2298
E-mail: info@dunitz.co.uk
Website: http://www.dunitz.co.uk

Although every effort has been made to ensure that drug doses and other information are presented accurately in this publication, the ultimate responsibility rests with the prescribing physician. Neither the publishers nor the authors can be held responsible for errors or for any consequences arising from the use of information contained herein. For detailed prescribing information or instructions on the use of any product or procedure discussed herein, please consult the prescribing information or instructional material issued by the manufacturer.

A CIP record for this book is available from the British Library.

ISBN 1 84184 088 2

Distributed in the USA by
Fulfilment Center
Taylor & Francis
10650 Tobben Drive
Independence, KY 41051, USA
Toll Free Tel: +1-800-634-7064
E-mail: taylorandfrancis@thomsonlearning.com

Distributed in Canada by
Taylor & Francis
74 Rolark Drive
Scarborough
Ontario M1R 4G2, Canada
Toll Free Tel: +1-877-226-2237
E-mail: tal_fran@istar.ca

Distributed in the rest of the world by
Thomson Publishing Services
Cheriton House
North Way, Andover
Hampshire SP10 5BE, UK
Tel: +44 (0)1264 332424
E-mail: salesorder.tandf@thomsonpublishingservices.co.uk

Printed and bound in Spain by E.G. Zure SA.

Preface

Chronic viral hepatitis affects over 500 million people worldwide and leads to cirrhosis and liver cell cancer in a large proportion of infected individuals. The optimal management of those who are infected requires close collaboration between the pathologist, who identifies the grade and stage of the disease, and the physician who implements therapy. In this succinct guide, two experienced teachers present a complete guide to the investigation and management of chronic viral hepatitis. The authors outline the mechanisms underlying persistent viral infection and go on to describe the epidemiology, virology and diagnosis of chronic viral hepatitis before outlining a comprehensive guide to modern, biopsy-based management. We describe the use of the latest therapies, including the pegylated interferons, and this well-written book will be of value to hepatologists, gastroenterologists and infectious disease physicians who care for patients with chronic viral hepatitis.

Graham R Foster
Robert D Goldin
London

Abbreviations

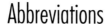

AFP	alpha-fetoprotein
AIDS	acquired immunodeficiency syndrome
cccDNA	covalently closed circular DNA
CT	computed tomography
DNA	deoxyribonucleic acid
HAI	histological activity index
HBcAg	hepatitis B virus core antigen
HBeAg	hepatitis B e antigen
HBIg	hepatitis B immunoglobulin
HBsAg	hepatitis B virus surface antigen
HIV	human immunodeficiency virus
HLA	human leucocyte antigen
IL	interleukin
iu	international units
MRI	magnetic resonance imaging
NS	non-structural
PCR	polymerase chain reaction
RNA	ribonucleic acid

Chronic viral hepatitis – persistence, prevalence and transmission

1

Most adult humans suffer from at least four or five viral infections every year. In almost all cases antiviral defence mechanisms recognize and rapidly eliminate the virus so that the illness is usually trivial and short-lasting.

Infection with the chronic hepatotropic viruses is very different – these pathogens commonly evade the antiviral defence systems and cause a long-lasting, persistent infection. The prolonged nature of the infection ensures that every infected person has ample opportunity to transmit the virus to others, allowing many millions of people world-wide to become infected. Three viruses commonly cause chronic hepatitis – hepatitis B virus, hepatitis C virus and delta virus. Virologically, these three pathogens are remarkably different but all have developed mechanisms that allow persistent infection, and overall they infect over 500 million people world-wide.

Mechanisms of persistence: how do hepatotropic viruses cause chronic infection?

Most viral infections are transient – after infection the virus is rapidly eliminated by the combined effects of the innate and the acquired immune systems. To cause persistent infection a virus must avoid the host defences and the hepatotropic viruses have developed elaborate strategies to achieve this.

Avoiding the innate immune system

The innate immune system is the first line of defence against pathogens. It consists of an arsenal of preformed circulating proteins as well as a series of cellular receptors that, when activated, trigger the release of proinflammatory cytokines. The circulating proteins of the innate immune system, such as mannose-binding lectin, bind to and neutralize infecting pathogens. These proteins play a key role in eliminating bacteria but they probably play a relatively minor role in combating viral infection. The surface receptors of the innate system are members of the TOLL-like family of receptors. These are activated by bacterial products and they activate the release of cytokines, such as tumour

necrosis factor (TNF) and interleukin (IL-1), which lead to inflammation and the activation of macrophages and lymphocytes. Again, activation of the TOLL-like receptors is an important component of the host defence against bacteria, but it is probably only of minor importance in the elimination of viruses.

The most important innate antiviral defence system is the type I interferons. These interferons are a family of closely related cytokines that consists of 12 interferon-alpha subtypes, one interferon-beta subtype and one interferon-omega subtype. These interferons are rapidly produced by virally infected cells and, once released, they bind to cell surface receptors and induce the production of a large number of proteins that inhibit viral replication.

The functions of some of the proteins that are induced by the type I interferons are well characterized, but no function has yet been identified for many of them. Some of the interferon-inducible proteins are produced in an inactive form and are activated by viral products. For example, type I interferons induce the production of a protein kinase known as 'PKR'. In the presence of a replicating RNA virus, this protein is activated by double-stranded RNA, and the activated kinase inhibits cellular protein production, thereby leading to suppression of viral replication. Other interferon-inducible proteins inhibit the replication of other viruses (e.g. the Mx protein inhibits the replication of the influenza virus), and it is assumed that many of the hundred or so interferon-induced proteins identified to date inhibit the replication of specific viruses, although not all of the targets have been identified (Table 1.1). It is not yet known which of the interferon-inducible proteins inhibit the replication of the hepatotropic viruses. The antiviral effects of the type I interferons are shown schematically in Figure 1.1.

In addition to activating an antiviral state in cells exposed to viruses, the type I interferons have immunomodulatory effects. They facilitate immune recognition of virally infected cells by increasing the cell surface expression of the human leucocyte antigen (HLA) class I antigens. These proteins present viral antigens to the cells of the immune system (see page 6) and thereby facilitate the immune-mediated destruction of virally infected cells. The type I interferons also facilitate the activation of the Th1 subset of helper T cells by increasing the expression of the IL-12 receptor and thereby increasing responsiveness to this cytokine.

Since the type I interferons are potent inhibitors of viral replication, viruses that lead to prolonged infection must have developed mechanisms to overcome the effects of these interferons, and many viruses encode proteins that inhibit the interferon system in some way.

In the case of the hepatitis B virus, two proteins are involved in this inhibition – the core protein has been been shown to inhibit the production of interferon, and the polymerase protein has been shown to inhibit its effects.

In the case of the hepatitis C virus, the NS5A and E2 proteins reduce the effects of interferon by inhibiting the antiviral kinase, PKR. However, not all hepatitis C NS5A proteins are inhibitory, and attempts have been made to correlate the clinical response to interferon with the sequence of the NS5A protein. To date such studies have been inconclusive, but it is possible that future studies will lead to the identification of 'interferon-sensitive' sequences and 'interferon-resistant' sequences, and it is foreseeable that such information will be used to guide therapeutic decisions.

Avoiding the acquired immune system

The acquired immune system provides

Table 1.1
Proteins that are induced by interferon-alpha. Several hundred proteins are induced when the type I interferons bind to the cell surface receptor, and only a few well-studied examples are listed here.

Protein	Function	Comments
PKR	Inhibits the replication of viruses that contain double-stranded RNA by blocking protein translation	Activated by double-stranded RNA
2'5' oligoadenylate synthetase	Inhibits the replication of viruses that contain double-stranded RNA by inducing its degradation	Activated by double-stranded RNA
Mx	Inhibits the replication of influenza virus	
HLA class I antigens	Presents foreign peptides to lymphocytes	
IL-12 receptor beta chain	Essential for response to IL-12	Sensitizes naïve T cells to the effects of IL-12 and thereby allows the development of a mature T cell response
6-16	Unknown	Used to study the interferon signal transduction pathway
ISG 15	Unknown	Used to study the interferon signal transduction pathway
9-27	Unknown	
ISG 54	Unknown	

Figure 1.1

Antiviral effects of the type I interferons. The type I interferon (usually interferon-alpha or interferon-beta) binds to the two components of the interferon receptor (A). Binding and dimerization activates a complex signal transduction pathway that involves sequential activation of a series of phosphoproteins (known as the JAKs and STATs) (B). This process ultimately leads to the production of a large number of interferon-inducible genes (C), including Mx, 2'5' oligoadenylate synthetase and the protein kinase PKR. The PKR protein is produced in an inactive form and is activated by double stranded RNA produced by infecting viruses (D). The activated kinase inhibits protein translation (by phosphorylating the translation initiation factor eIF2-alpha. The inhibition of protein translation prevents further viral replication (E).

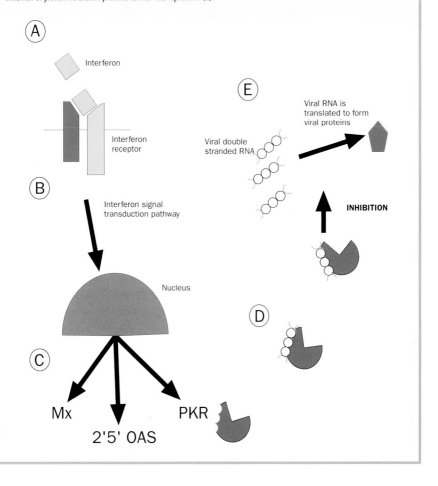

long-lasting, pathogen-specific immunity and involves the production of antibodies and the generation of antiviral T cells. Circulating antibodies can neutralize virions, and they can bind to viral proteins that are expressed on the surface of cells and, by fixing complement, lyse them. Different classes of antibody are typically produced during different stages of an infection – initially IgM-type antibodies are produced but later IgG-type antibodies predominate. The identification of the type of circulating antibody may help to distinguish acute from chronic infection.

Antiviral T cells are activated T lymphocytes that inhibit viral replication. Two groups of T lymphocytes may act as antiviral T cells : CD4-positive 'helper' T cells and CD8-positive 'cytotoxic' T cells. The CD4-positive T cells that inhibit viral replication belong to the Th1 group of CD4-positive T cells, and they inhibit viral replication by local production of antiviral cytokines (such as interferon-gamma). The cytotoxic T cells (CD8-positive T cells) inhibit viral replication by lysing virally infected cells, either by producing lytic proteins or by activating endogenous apoptotic pathways by Fas/FasL interactions. For both of these antiviral T cells close contact with the virally infected cell is essential for activity, and the activated T cells recognize virally infected cells only when the infected cells express viral antigens on their surface. Surface expression of viral proteins by HLA class I antigens involves:

- cleavage of viral proteins by a collection of cellular enzymes (the proteosome);
- transport of the peptides into the endoplasmic reticulum by transporter (TAP) proteins; and
- cell surface presentation in association with HLA class I antigens.

The development and activation of antiviral lymphocytes is a complex process that involves:

- uptake of viral antigens by dendritic cells;
- presentation of viral peptides to helper T cells; and
- interaction between helper T cells and effector T cells, which leads to the generation of antiviral T cells.

The activated antiviral T cells recognize virally infected cells when the target cell expresses viral antigens in the context of HLA class I antigens on their surface. This presentation of viral antigens to T cells is enhanced by type I interferons, which up-regulate HLA class I antigens (see page 3). The development of a cellular antiviral immune response is illustrated in Figure 1.2.

Figure 1.2
Generation of cellular immune responses. Viral proteins from infected hepatocytes are ingested by dendritic cells (or the hepatocytes are themselves phagocytosed) (A, B). The immature dendritic cells process the viral proteins (B) and migrate to the local lymph nodes, where they mature into 'professional' antigen-presenting cells (C). The mature antigen-presenting cells present the processed antigens on their surface in association with HLA class II antigens (C). Circulating T cells that recognize the foreign antigens activate (license) the antigen-presenting cells (D) and the activated antigen-presenting cells then interact with other lymphocytes (including cytotoxic T cells – CD8+ cells) and activate them (E). The activated T cells (both helper T cells (CD4+ T cells) and cytotoxic (CD8+ T cells)) migrate to the liver, where they identify infected cells that express foreign antigens on their surface in association with HLA class I antigens. The activated lymphocytes either inhibit viral replication, via local production of cytokines (Th1 cells) or induce lysis of the infected cells (CD8+ cells).

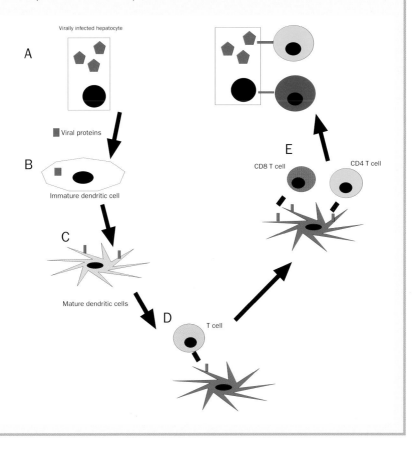

The development of an effective antiviral cellular immune response requires activation of the Th1 subset of helper T cells. Activation of the other helper T cell subset (Th2, CD4-positive T cells) inhibits activation of the Th1 cells and probably facilitates viral persistence.[1]

The factors that determine whether a Th1 or a Th2 T cell response develops are therefore critical in determining the outcome of a viral infection; at present, our understanding of these crucial control mechanisms is incomplete and little is known about the way in which Th1 and Th2 responses are regulated.

Persistent viral infection is associated with avoidance of both arms of the immune system. The mechanisms of persistent viral infection are not completely understood but some general features are beginning to emerge. Mutation of viral

proteins is a powerful avoidance strategy used by many viruses. Antibodies and circulating T cells recognize and bind to small, specific regions within viral proteins (epitopes). If these sequences change then the antibody or T cell can no longer recognize the viral protein and hence the virus can evade the antiviral defences. The hepatitis C virus uses this approach to avoid neutralizing antibodies – the envelope protein mutates at a high rate – and it is thought that cytotoxic T cells can be avoided by changes in other viral proteins. The hepatitis B virus avoids immune attack based on the hepatitis B 'e' antigen (HBeAg) by mutating so that this protein is not produced at all (see page 73).

Viruses can also avoid the immune response by preventing activation of the system in the first instance. This effect can be specific or non-specific – the notorious human immunodeficiency virus (HIV) kills all immune responses by killing T cells, but the hepatotropic viruses are much more subtle and influence the immune system in multiple, albeit ill-understood, ways. The hepatitis B virus produces a small protein (HBeAg), which crosses the placenta and induces tolerance to itself, and related hepatitis B proteins. Because the immune system has come into contact with the protein in

[1] Th1 helper T cells are characterized by the production of proinflammatory cytokines such as IL-2 and interferon-gamma. Th2 helper T cells produce IL-4, IL-5 and IL-10, and these cytokines facilitate the production of antibodies and inhibit the development of Th1 cells. Hence Th1 cells predominantly assist in the development of cellular immune responses – important for elimination of viruses – and Th2 cells play a major role in the development of humoral and eosinophilic immune responses.

early life, the immune system believes the protein to be 'self' and is therefore unable to mount an effective immune response. The hepatitis C virus can also inhibit the generation of an appropriate immune response, and infection of dendritic cells is one mechanism which may be used by this virus.

Prevalence of viral hepatitis

Hepatitis C

> *Throughout the world chronic infection with the hepatitis C virus is common, and the World Health Organization estimates that over 170 million people are infected.*

The prevalence of hepatitis C virus infection varies between different countries, and different regions within the same country may have markedly different prevalence rates (Table 1.2).

For example, in some Italian villages the prevalence may be as high as 20% whereas the prevalence in other parts of Italy is no greater than 2%.

In Europe as a whole, the prevalence of chronic hepatitis C virus infection increases along a north–south axis, with the northern, Scandinavian countries having a low prevalence (less than 0.5%) and the southern, Mediterranean countries having a higher prevalence, approaching 2%. The reasons for this variation are unclear.

The prevalence of chronic hepatitis C virus infection in the USA is similar to that in southern Europe (1.8%).

The prevalence in Africa is probably a little higher and is estimated to be around 2–5%.

In the Middle East, infection is common and affects between 1 and 12% of the population. The prevalence is particularly high in Egypt, where infection rates as high as 20% have been found. This unusually high prevalence is believed to be due to the use of unsterilized needles during therapy for schistosomiasis, but this has not been formally proven.

Transmission of the hepatitis C virus

> *Hepatitis C is a blood-borne virus that is transmitted by blood-to-blood contact – the virus is relatively difficult to pass on, and exposure to fresh blood or relatively large amounts of stored blood seems to be required to transmit the infection.*

Table 1.2
Prevalence of chronic hepatitis C infection in selected areas. Note that widespread epidemiological studies have not yet been performed, and the true prevalence and distribution of this virus have not yet been elucidated

Continent	Country	Prevalence (%)	Comments
Europe	Sweden	0.3	Typical prevalence seen in northern Europe
	Italy (general)	2	
	Italy (Bari province)	26	Unusual cluster of cases
	Sardinia	7	
	Spain	0.8	
North America	USA	1.8	Based on a large, community survey
Africa	Cameroon	6.8	
	Egypt	26.6	

Because of the mode of transmission of hepatitis C virus, infection is common in those who have used intravenous drugs and in those who have shared injecting paraphernalia; it is also found in people who have received contaminated blood or blood products. In the developed world, transmission via blood products was curtailed in the early 1990s, when screening of all donated blood for hepatitis C began, and this route of transmission is now exceedingly rare.

The majority of new cases of hepatitis C virus infection in the developed world are now found in people who misuse drugs.

Intravenous drug use carries the highest risk but nasal ingestion of cocaine (by snorting) may also transmit the virus, probably via blood-stained straws or other equipment.

Transmission of hepatitis C by contaminated blood or medical equipment is, sadly, still common in the underdeveloped world and, in many countries, this remains the major route of infection.

In addition to the common routes of transmission, a number of other modes of infection exist. Maternal–fetal transmission is rare and occurs in less than 5% of deliveries from mothers who are infected with hepatitis C. The risk of maternal–fetal transmission is increased if the mother has a high level of viraemia, and this is common in patients who are immunosuppressed. Hence maternal–fetal transmission is much more common in patients who are infected with both hepatitis C and HIV. Sexual transmission of hepatitis C is uncommon, although not impossible, and the prevalence of chronic hepatitis C virus infection in promiscuous people is only slightly greater than in those with few sexual partners. Percutaneous exposure with unsterilized piercing equipment (e.g. during body piercing or tattooing) may transmit the virus but this is now uncommon. Risk factors for chronic hepatitis C virus infection are shown in Table 1.3.

Medical staff may be infected with the hepatitis C virus via needle stick injuries from infected patients. This is extremely rare and recipients of needle stick injuries should be reassured that infection is unlikely. To confirm that infection has not occurred, a sample of the recipient's blood should be examined for the presence of the virus after 3 months (hepatitis C virus polymerase chain reaction test), and the absence of infection should be confirmed after 6 months by serological assays (hepatitis C virus antibody tests). It is also wise to perform a baseline test immediately after exposure to look for antibodies against hepatitis C to confirm that the person is not already infected.

Infection of patients by infected health-care personnel is extremely uncommon, but a few incidents of transmission have occurred in which an infected surgeon has infected a patient during an operation. Whether all surgeons should be screened for hepatitis C and barred from invasive procedures if found to be positive is a sensitive issue that is currently under consideration. Screening all surgeons and preventing those who are infected with hepatitis C from operating would prevent a very small number of transmissions, but the costs and the problems associated with reducing the number of operating surgeons would be considerable and many people feel that the disadvantages outweigh the benefits.

Prevention of hepatitis C virus infection
At present there is no effective vaccine against hepatitis C virus, and prevention of infection therefore relies on:

- screening of blood products for the virus; and
- prevention of transmission among active drug users by appropriate education and provision of clean injecting paraphernalia.

Table 1.3
Risk factors for infection with the hepatitis C virus

Risk factor	Comment
Intravenous drug use	Most common mode of transmission in the developed world. The period of drug use may have ended many years before presentation
Other drug use (e.g. snorting cocaine)	Rare mode of transmission
Blood or blood product transfusion	Common in those transfused before 1990, but now very rare in developed countries
Incarceration	Infection is common in prisoners, probably as a result of drug abuse leading to incarceration or drug abuse in prison
Hospital therapy	Very rare mode of acquisition in the developed world. Remains a common route of transmission in many underdeveloped countries. Some medical procedures (e.g. dialysis) carry a very high risk and stringent precautions are required to prevent transmission
Infected mother	Risk is less than 5% unless the parent is also infected with HIV
Infected family member	Very low risk. Family members should not share blood-stained devices such as razors and toothbrushes
Body piercing	Very small risk
Promiscuity	Very low risk

It is important to recognize that intravenous drug users may transmit the virus by contact with contaminated injecting paraphernalia (such as tourniquets, spoons etc – known colloquially as 'the works'), and therefore simple provision of clean needles and advice not to share needles may not be sufficient to prevent the spread of hepatitis C. Injecting drug users must be advised not to share any item of injecting equipment.

Hepatitis B

Hepatitis B virus is an extremely common virus throughout the world. It is endemic in many populations, ranging from the Inuit in Alaska to the Polynesian islanders in the south Pacific. In endemic parts of the world – Africa, the Far East and the Amazon basin – up to 80% of the population have evidence of exposure to hepatitis B virus and up to 20% are actively infected. In the developed world hepatitis B is uncommon and the prevalence varies from 5 to 10% in the Mediterranean countries to less than 2% in northern Europe and the USA. The prevalence of hepatitis B virus infection around the world is shown in Figure 1.3.

Transmission of the hepatitis B virus

The hepatitis B virus is extremely infectious and is readily transmitted by blood-to-blood contact.

In endemic areas, hepatitis B virus is mainly transmitted within families – mothers infect their infants in early life and the infected children infect other children during rough play.

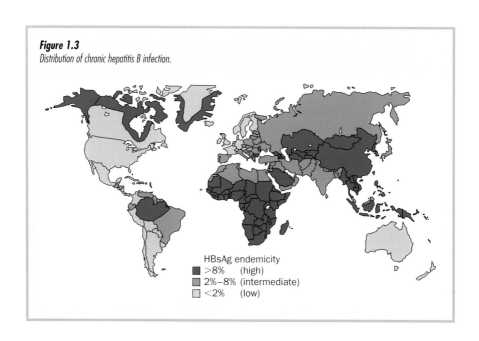

Figure 1.3
Distribution of chronic hepatitis B infection.

HBsAg endemicity
■ >8%   (high)
■ 2%–8% (intermediate)
□ <2%   (low)

An interesting, but unexplained, observation is that in Asia transmission occurs from mothers to their infants during childbirth but in Africa the virus is passed on in early childhood. Many of these infected children go on to eliminate the virus and the persistence of viral antibodies is the only evidence of exposure; however, others go on to become chronically infected.

In areas of the world where hepatitis B is not endemic, the virus is easily transmitted to non-vaccinated people by close contact with those who are infected. In contrast to hepatitis C, the hepatitis B virus is very infectious and exposure to miniscule amounts of blood is sufficient to transmit the pathogen.

Sexual transmission occurs, and hepatitis B virus is more often found in those who are promiscuous, particularly in men who have sex with men.

The virus may be passed on by drug misuse but in many Western countries the virus has not become established in the drug-using community and hence relatively few intravenous drug users are infected.

Over the past few years the increase in young adults travelling to exotic holiday locations has led to an increase in hepatitis B virus infection in this group and teenagers with hepatitis B virus infection should be questioned carefully about recent sexual experiences abroad.

> *Medical staff are at high risk of infection with hepatitis B and all medical personnel should be vaccinated against the virus and should have regular determinations of their antibody titre.*

A circulating antibody titre of more than 1 in 100 is regarded as protective and if the titre falls to approaching this level a booster vaccination should be given. In medical personnel who do not respond to the current vaccine any needle stick injury from an infected patient should be reported immediately. The early (within 24 hours) administration of hepatitis B immunoglobulin (HBIg) at a dose of 500 iu by intramuscular injection may prevent transmission.

Health-care workers who are infected with hepatitis B virus may transmit the virus to patients during invasive procedures. Those who are most likely to transmit the virus are:

- those who are HBeAg-positive; and
- those who are HBeAg-negative but have high levels of circulating virus.

In many countries such health-care workers are barred from performing exposure-prone invasive procedures. (The definition of 'high levels of circulating virus' differs from country to country. Some authorities consider 'high level' to be more than 10^5 copies/ml, whereas others regard 3×10^4 (the lowest level at which transmission has been documented) as 'high level'.)

Prevention of hepatitis B virus infection

> *Hepatitis B virus infection can be effectively prevented by vaccination.*

The surface antigen of hepatitis B is highly immunogenic and causes prolonged immunity in the majority of vaccinated people. The original hepatitis B vaccines were derived from the serum of patients who had partially eliminated the virus, but the current vaccines are derived from genetically engineered yeast; hence there is no risk of infection with other blood-borne pathogens during vaccination. Vaccination against hepatitis B virus is effective, but a few individuals are unresponsive to the current vaccine. For these people, protection is not possible at present; however, new vaccines that may overcome the problem are being developed.

There is ongoing debate as to whether all hepatitis B vaccine recipients should be tested for the presence of antibodies and offered booster vaccinations at regular intervals. The current consensus is that such an approach is unnecessary (the anamnestic response to the first vaccination schedule should provide sufficient protection against further exposure), but in people at very high risk (e.g. medical personnel) it may be prudent to adopt a more cautious approach and maintain high titres of protective antibody, as outlined above. The introduction of global vaccination in parts of the world where hepatitis B virus infection is common (e.g. Italy and Taiwan) has led to a fall in the prevalence of hepatocellular carcinoma, indicating that vaccination is an effective means of reducing the mortality and morbidity of chronic hepatitis B virus infection.

Hepatitis delta

Infection with the delta virus is possible only in people who are also infected with hepatitis B virus. The delta virus may be contracted either simultaneously with the hepatitis B virus (co-infection) or later (superinfection). Hence the virus is common only in areas where hepatitis B is endemic. However, not all areas that have a high prevalence of hepatitis B have a high rate of hepatitis delta superinfection. For example, the virus is rare in most of southern Africa but common in Venezuela and some Mediterranean countries.

The delta virus is a blood-borne virus that may be transmitted by parenteral contract. In developed countries the virus is normally associated with intravenous drug use although in some countries (in particular Romania) nosocomial transmission from contaminated medical equipment has led to a high prevalence in some populations. In South America, epidemics of the virus with a high mortality occur infrequently, but the route of transmission in these outbreaks is not yet clear. Sexual transmission of the delta virus is uncommon.

Prevention of infection with the delta virus relies on effective prevention of hepatitis B virus infection by vaccination.

Other hepatotropic viruses

A small number of patients develop a chronic hepatitis that appears to be transmitted by blood or blood products but is not due to one of the currently identified hepatitis viruses – this is known as non-A–E hepatitis. The virus responsible for this infection has not been identified but a number of possible aetiological agents have been proposed.

These include hepatitis G virus (also known as GBV-C) and the transfusion transmitted virus (TTV). A number of epidemiological studies have shown that these agents are unlikely to be the cause of most cases of non-A–E hepatitis, and it is likely that these viruses do not cause significant liver disease.

Further reading

Koziel M. The role of immune responses in the pathogenesis of hepatitis C virus infection. *J Viral Hep* 1997; **4S1**: 31–41.

Mart EE, Alter MJ. Epidemiology of viral hepatitis: an overview. *Semin Virol* 1993; **4**: 273–83.

Pestka S, Langer T, Zoon K, Samuel C. Interferons and their actions. *Annu Rev Biochem* 1987; **56**: 727–77.

WHO. Global surveillance and control of hepatitis C. *J Viral Hep* 1999; **6**: 35–47.

Questions

1. Regarding chronic hepatitis B virus infection in Africa:
   A. Over 80% of the population are actively infected

B. Maternal–fetal transmission usually occurs *in utero*

C. Sexual transmission does not occur

D. Chronic infection has a good prognosis

E. Co-infection with hepatitis C is common

2. Regarding chronic hepatitis C virus infection:

A. It is common in prostitutes who do not use drugs

B. Transmission between intravenous drug users can be eliminated by needle exchange programmes

C. It is rarely passed from mothers to their children

D. It may be passed on from infected health-care personnel

E. Transmission can be prevented by vaccination

3. Infection with the delta virus:

A. Can be prevented by successful vaccination against hepatitis B virus

B. Is always associated with chronic hepatitis C virus infection

C. Never causes severe disease

D. Is common in northern Europe

E. May cause outbreaks of hepatitis

4. The type I interferons:

A. Inhibit the replication of the hepatitis B virus by the effects of the protein kinase PKR

B. Are induced within a few hours of viral infection

C. May be inhibited by viral infection

D. Are of little importance in eliminating viral infections

E. Enhance immune recognition of virally infected cells

Answers

Question 1

A. False – active infection with viraemia affects no more than 20% of the population

B. False – maternal–fetal transmission occurs during delivery or early life

C. False

D. False

E. False

Question 2

A. False – sexual transmission is rare and infection in sex workers is unusual unless they also abuse drugs

B. False – the virus can be transmitted on injecting paraphernalia

C. True

D. True

E. False

Question 3

A. True
B. False – it is associated with hepatitis B virus infection
C. False – it typically causes more severe disease
D. False
E. True

Question 4

A. False – it is not yet clear how interferon inhibits the replication of hepatitis B virus, but PKR, which is active against double-stranded RNA viruses, is unlikely to be involved
B. True
C. True
D. False – they are crucial, and genetically engineered mice that do not respond to interferon die rapidly from normally trivial viral infections
E. True

Hepatitis C – virology, natural history and pathology

2

Since its discovery in 1989 the hepatitis C virus has been extensively studied by both academic and commercial research groups. However, progress has been relatively slow and our current knowledge remains fragmentary. The natural history of the disease caused by the hepatitis C virus (formally known as non-A–non-B hepatitis) has proved difficult to study because there is no appropriate small animal model. Hence, much of our present understanding about this virus and its associated disease is likely to change over the next few years.

Hepatitis C – the virus

The hepatitis C virus has not yet been visualized and there is no *in vitro* replication system that allows a full analysis of the viral replication cycle. Much of our current information is therefore derived from inference and speculation based on comparisons with other viruses that are easier to study. This information has been supplemented with data that are derived from studies of the individual viral proteins, but it is likely that a full understanding of the replication cycle of hepatitis C virus will be available only when *in vitro* replication systems have been developed.

Viral structure

The hepatitis C virus genome consists of a single strand of RNA that is directly processed to produce the viral proteins (i.e. it is a positive-strand RNA virus). The genome is very similar to viruses in the Flaviviridae family (such as the yellow fever and dengue viruses) and, by analogy, the functions of the different regions of the hepatitis C virus genome have been identified. These are shown in Figure 2.1.

In common with many RNA viruses, the hepatitis C virus mutates at a very high rate. This means that in any infected patient there are multiple different viruses, each differing by a few nucleotides, and one or two amino acids – in other words, the virus exists as a population of closely related but different viral species (quasispecies). Over time some of these different viral species are more successful and become dominant, so that the viral population changes. It is estimated that the dominant viral sequence changes every few weeks. These changes may help the hepatitis C virus to avoid the immune system (see page 6).

Figure 2.1
The diagram shows a schematic representation of the proteins encoded by the hepatitis C virus genome. The genome consists of a non-coding region (the 5' untranslated region (UTR) linked to a coding region that encodes the proteins illustrated in the figure. At the 5' end of the virus the RNA encodes the structural proteins (core (C) and the envelope proteins E1 and E2). The function of the small p7 protein is unknown. Following the structural proteins are the non-structural proteins (the NS proteins). NS2 is a protease that cleaves the viral polyprotein, NS3 is a complex protein that encodes a helicase and a protease and NS4A is a co-factor that binds to and activates NS3. NS5 is split into two proteins – NS5A is of unknown function but may inhibit the cellular response to interferon and NS5B is an RNA polymerase that replicates the viral genome.

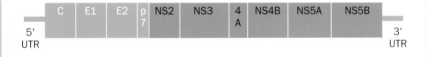

It is likely that the high mutation rate of the hepatitis C virus will make it difficult to develop a single antiviral drug or vaccine that will eliminate or prevent infection – as with HIV, multiple drugs will probably be required to treat hepatitis C virus infection successfully.

Since the genomic sequence of the hepatitis C virus changes every few weeks it is not surprising to find that every patient is infected with a slightly different version of the virus and no two people have an identical viral population.

However, people who are initially infected with the same virus will develop a viral population that is related, and by examining the sequence of the viruses one can examine the possibility that two people infected each other. These types of analysis are of obvious forensic value.

Within the hepatitis C virus there are regions that are reasonably stable and change relatively little (these include the non-coding regions and the hepatitis C virus core protein). The slow evolution of these conserved regions has differed in different geographical regions and has led to the evolution of different

strains of hepatitis C virus, known as genotypes.

At least six genotypes are now recognized (Table 2.1). All of the different genotypes appear to have a similar effect on the liver (i.e. disease progression is similar for all of them) but the response to therapy is influenced by genotype, and different durations of treatment are required to treat the different genotypes (see page 56). These genotypes can be subdivided (e.g. genotype 1 has been subdivided into type 1a and type 1b) but this is not of value in clinical practice.

Replication of the hepatitis C virus

Our knowledge of the replication of the hepatitis C virus is still incomplete. The information that is currently available is being used to develop new antiviral agents and it is likely that the currently identified drug targets will lead to novel therapeutic agents in the foreseeable future.

The hepatitis C virus enters an hepatocyte by binding to a specific cell surface receptor. The regions within the envelope protein that interact with the receptor have not been identified, but they are probably encoded by the E1 protein or the

Table 2.1
Genotypes of the hepatitis C virus and their main characteristics

Genotype	Distribution	Response to interferon and ribavirin therapy	Comments
1	World-wide	Poor – 48 weeks of therapy are required	Most common genotype in Europe, USA and Japan
2	World-wide	Good – 24 weeks of therapy required	
3	World-wide	Good – 24 weeks of therapy required	Common in drug users in the developed world
4	Middle East	Poor - 48 weeks of therapy are probably required, but few data are available	
5	Far East	Unknown	
6	South Africa	Unknown	

E2 protein, or possibly both. A complete understanding of the interaction between the hepatitis C virus and its receptor will allow predictions of crucial, invariate regions of the envelope protein to be derived. This will greatly facilitate vaccine designs, since vaccines targeted against these regions are unlikely to lead to the development of vaccine escape mutants. The cell membrane tetraspanin protein, CD81, may play a role in the entry of hepatitis C virus into cells; however, the details of this are not yet clear, and other, as yet unidentified cellular, proteins are also involved.

Following entry into the cell the hepatitis C genome is translated by host ribosomes to produce a single large protein, the polyprotein. The 5′ untranslated region of the hepatitis C virus plays a key role in this process and, since this region is highly conserved between different viral isolates, it may be possible to develop drugs that bind to this region and inhibit viral translation.

The polyprotein that is produced by translation of the hepatitis C virus genome is cleaved and processed to form a replication complex that associates with the endoplasmic reticulum. Cleavage of the hepatitis C polyprotein involves a number of proteases, including the non-structural (NS) proteins of the virus, NS2 and the NS3–4. The viral proteases from other viruses have been successfully inhibited by compounds that are therapeutically valuable, and hence the protease of hepatitis C is an attractive target for drug development. Sadly attempts to develop hepatitis C protease inhibitors have, to date, been unsuccessful.

Cleavage of the viral polyprotein releases and activates other viral proteins. The key proteins involved in the replication of the viral genome are the helicase protein (encoded by the NS3 region) and the polymerase protein (encoded by the NS5 region). These two proteins lead to the production of new hepatitis C viral RNA strands. Again, these viral proteins are attractive targets for novel antiviral agents.

The newly formed viral RNA strands are packaged into novel viral particles and released by mechanisms that are, as yet, poorly understood. The bovine diarrhoea virus, which is a closely related virus, is released from cells only after extensive glycosylation, and inhibiting this process inhibits the release of the virus. Since the envelope proteins of the hepatitis C virus are also glycosylated, it is possible that drugs that inhibit glycosylation may have activity against hepatitis C virus – this approach is under investigation.

Natural history of hepatitis C virus infection

Infection with the hepatitis C virus occasionally causes an acute hepatitis, in which the patient becomes overtly jaundiced with markedly raised serum transaminases.

> *Acute hepatitis caused by hepatitis C virus infection presentation is rare, and inapparent chronic infection lasting for decades is the most common form of hepatitis C virus infection. A small minority develop an icteric illness that leads to chronic anicteric hepatitis C.*

Chronic infection with the hepatitis C virus leads to a disease whose outcome is extremely variable. Most patients are unknowingly infected and are asymptomatic at the time of infection.

A small proportion (20%) of patients clear the virus and remain persistently non-viraemic with normal liver function tests. Exposure to the virus in these patients can be inferred from the presence of antibodies against the virus in the absence of detectable viraemia. Recurrence of viraemia in such patients has not been reported and is unlikely, although profound immunosuppression might, in theory, lead to reactivation.

For the 80% of exposed patients who develop a persistent infection spontaneous clearance is rare, and patients who are hepatitis C viraemic 12 months after exposure are very unlikely to clear the virus without therapy.

Some patients are infected with the hepatitis C virus for decades and, after 20–30 years, a liver biopsy shows minimal disease and no scarring. However, in others the disease progresses much more rapidly and within 10 years the liver inflammation leads to cirrhosis. For the majority of patients, the virus causes a slowly progressive fibrosis that leads to cirrhosis in more than three decades.

> *Overall the prognosis for patients with chronic hepatitis C virus infection is based on the '30–30 rule' – 30% will have cirrhosis after 30 years.*

It is widely assumed that the progression of fibrosis in chronic hepatitis C is linear and that the fibrosis slowly increases with time. This may not always be the case and in some patients quiescent disease may become active and the fibrosis may progress very rapidly. In others active disease with rapid scarring may slow, and some believe that the scarring may even reverse. Figure 2.2 illustrates the natural history of chronic hepatitis C virus infection.

> *The extent of the liver injury in chronic hepatitis C virus infection cannot be inferred from the standard liver function tests.*

In most patients with chronic infection the liver function tests fluctuate and may vary from normal to markedly raised over the space of a few days. Hence the only reliable way to assess this disease is to perform a liver biopsy. Even so, although liver function tests do not allow a reliable assessment of the extent of the liver damage in chronic hepatitis C virus infection they may be useful in assigning likelihood of liver damage – patients who have persistently

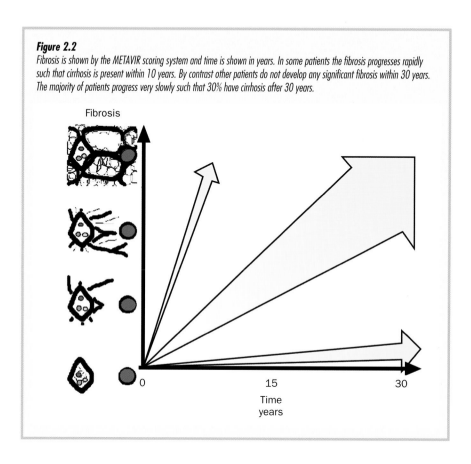

Figure 2.2
Fibrosis is shown by the METAVIR scoring system and time is shown in years. In some patients the fibrosis progresses rapidly such that cirrhosis is present within 10 years. By contrast other patients do not develop any significant fibrosis within 30 years. The majority of patients progress very slowly such that 30% have cirrhosis after 30 years.

normal liver function tests are more likely to have mild disease than those with markedly abnormal liver function tests, and *vice versa*.

The factors that influence the progression of chronic hepatitis C virus infection are still largely unknown. Patients who are

male and who contract the virus late in life (after the age of 40 years) tend to have more aggressive disease with more rapid development of the fibrosis, but in an individual patient it is impossible to predict the rate of progression of the disease. Excessive alcohol consumption (more than 40 g/day) accelerates the disease in all patients and should be avoided. Most authorities agree that even occasional alcohol consumption increases the rate of disease progression and is best avoided. Coexisting haemochromatosis or HIV infection are also associated with an increase in the rate of disease progression.

For patients with hepatitis C-related cirrhosis, the outlook is bleak. Every year a small percentage (around 5%) of such patients develop liver cell cancer and 2–3% develop decompensated liver disease. Without successful therapy or transplantation, death from cirrhosis and its complications is inevitable.

Pathology of hepatitis C

Histopathological features of chronic hepatitis C virus infection

A number of histopathological features have been described as being characteristic of hepatitis C virus infection (Table 2.2). The three most common of these are:

- the presence of portal lymphoid follicles and aggregates (Fig. 2.3);
- 'hepatitic' bile duct damage (Fig. 2.4); and
- fatty change (Fig. 2.5)

Lymphoid aggregates may be seen in other causes of chronic hepatitis, such as autoimmune hepatitis and even some cases of hepatitis B, as well as in primary biliary cirrhosis. Nevertheless they are much more common in hepatitis C, in which they tend to be better formed than in other conditions. In some cases of hepatitis C, the lymphoid aggregates have well-formed germinal centres, the presence of which can be confirmed by immunohistochemical staining. These germinal centres contain follicle centre cells and dendritic cells, and they are surrounded by a mantle zone that is rich in B cells, which is in turn surrounded by a zone that is rich in CD4-positive T cells. Well-formed lymphoid follicles are most often seen in cases with otherwise relatively inactive disease. The presence of lymphoid aggregates can be highlighted using a reticulin stain.

Table 2.2
Characteristic histological features in chronic hepatitis C

> Portal lymphoid follicles and aggregates
> 'Hepatitic' bile duct damage
> Fatty change
> Borderline interface hepatitis
> Prominent lobular inflammation

Figure 2.3
Liver biopsy from a case of chronic HCV with a characteristic portal tract lymphoid aggregate. There is no piecemeal necrosis/interface hepatitis.

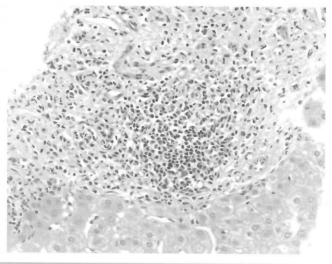

Figure 2.4
Liver biopsy from a case of chronic HCV with a characteristic bile duct damage (but not bile duct loss).

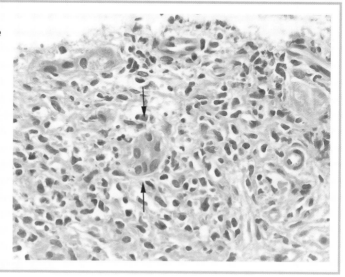

Figure 2.5
Liver biopsy from a case of chronic HCV with large droplet fatty change. Although this is characteristic of HCV, on its own this change is indistinguishable from alcohol induced liver damage.

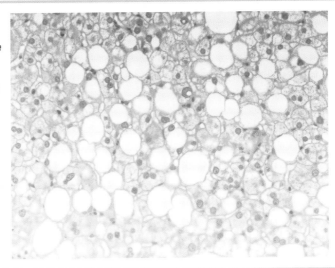

Figure 2.6
Liver biopsy from a patient with HCV who drinks excessively. The biopsy shows neutrophilic inflammation (within the enclosed area) and Mallory's hyaline within ballooned hepatocytes (one of which is arrowed). This indicates that alcohol is a significant contributing factor to this patients liver damage.

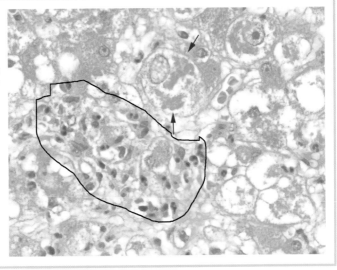

'Hepatitic' bile duct damage is also very common in hepatitis C virus infection. This damage is characterized by an inflammatory infiltrate that extends into the biliary epithelium, which itself shows degenerative changes, including cytoplasmic vacuolation and reactive nuclear changes (e.g. stratification and nuclear crowding). The key point is that there is no bile duct loss – bile duct loss in a patient with hepatitis C should initiate a search for another cause, such as primary sclerosing cholangitis. Canalicular cholestasis is also exceptionally uncommon in chronic hepatitis C virus infection, and its presence should prompt a search for an additional cause of liver disease – the most common are a drug-induced hepatitis and a superimposed acute viral hepatitis (most usually infection with hepatitis A virus).

Fatty change is common in hepatitis C virus infection, as it is in many liver diseases, including, of course, alcohol-induced liver disease. A relatively common question asked of pathologists is whether the liver damage seen in a biopsy from a patient with hepatitis C who also drinks alcohol is due mainly to the infection or to the alcohol intake. The presence, distribution and severity of the fatty change is of no help in making this decision. The presence of significant alcohol-induced liver injury can only be made when the biopsy shows:

- ballooning degeneration of hepatocytes with Mallory's hyaline stain (Fig. 2.6);
- a neutrophilic infiltrate (see Fig. 2.6); and
- pericellular fibrosis (Fig. 2.7).

Neither Mallory's hyaline nor pericellular fibrosis are seen in cases of uncomplicated hepatitis C (despite claims to the contrary).

> *The diagnosis of hepatitis C virus infection is rarely, if ever, made on the basis of liver biopsy.*

In rare cases, the presence of one or (more significantly) more of these three changes in a patient in whom hepatitis C virus infection is unsuspected should suggest the need for the serology to be rechecked. This is particularly true in acute hepatitis C, in which serology is not always reliable. It should be noted that in cases of acute hepatitis C virus infection these three characteristic histological are often seen. In patients with coexisting hepatitis C and hepatitis B features of both diseases are seen.

It is typical of hepatitis C virus infection that the degree of interface hepatitis is

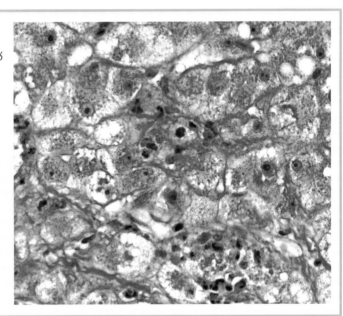

Figure 2.7
Liver biopsy from the same patient as Fig. 2.6 showing pericellular fibrosis which is also characteristic of alcohol induced liver damage (trichrome stain).

usually mild and the degree of lobular inflammation is often greater than that seen in hepatitis B virus infection (Figs 2.8–2.11). This is one of the reasons why the classification of chronic hepatitis into chronic persistent hepatitis and chronic active hepatitis, which depends entirely on the presence or absence of interface hepatitis, has fallen into disuse. Prominent acidophilic degeneration of hepatocytes that leads to the formation of apoptotic bodies is characteristic of hepatitis C. The lobular inflammation can take the form of a widespread sinusoidal infiltrate that is similar to the picture seen with Epstein–Barr virus. Granulomas are more common in chronic hepatitis C than in chronic hepatitis B. However, if a granuloma is seen in a patient with hepatitis C virus infection, every effort should be made to exclude other causes of hepatic granulomas (e.g. tuberculosis, sarcoidosis). Hepatocyte dysplasia may also be seen, especially in cirrhotic livers (see page 150).

Figure 2.8
Liver biopsy from a
patient with HCV showing
apoptosis which is a
common form of liver cell
damage in this form of
hepatitis. It is uncommon
in HBV except when
there is co-existent HDV.

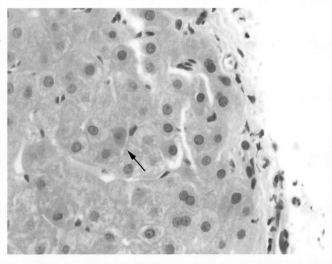

Figure 2.9
The same case as in
Fig. 2.8 with a sinusoidal
pattern of lymphoid
infiltration (arrowed)
which is seen in HCV and
also in infectious
mononucleosis.

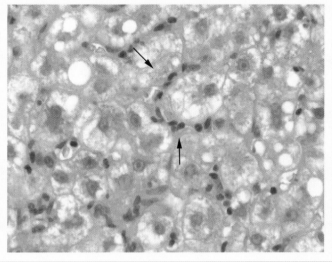

Figure 2.10
Liver biopsy from a patient with HCV with irregularity of the limiting plate (i.e. the interface between the connective tissue of the portal tract and the hepatocytes in the lobules) indicative of interface hepatitis (piecemeal necrosis).

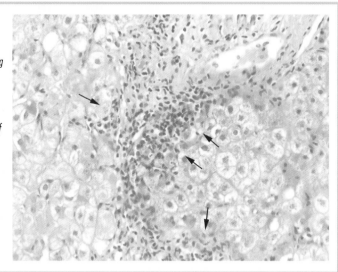

Figure 2.11
Liver biopsy from the same patient as in Fig. 2.10 showing, at a higher power, a periportal hepatocyte (arrowed) surrounding by lymphocytes and which shows degenerative features. This is the defining feature of interface hepatitis (piecemeal necrosis).

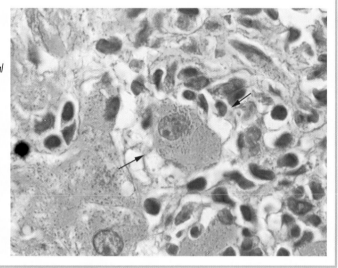

Immunohistochemical staining has no role to play in the routine assessment of liver biopsies in patients with hepatitis C because no commercially available antibody has been shown to work reliably on formalin-fixed, paraffin-embedded tissue. *In situ* PCR to detect the viral RNA in tissue is also not used in clinical practice. As is the case with hepatitis B, PCR on liver tissue may be positive even if it has been negative in the serum.

Given the frequency with which patients with hepatitis C undergo liver biopsy it is not surprising that some of them are also found to have another type of liver disease. The most common of these are:

- alcohol-induced liver disease; and
- genetic haemochromatosis.

The interpretation of alcohol-induced changes in patients with hepatitis C has been discussed above. To assess the degree of iron overload, and its distribution, it is necessary for all liver biopsies to be stained specifically for iron (Perl's Prussian blue reaction) (Figs 2.12 and 2.13).

In genetic haemochromatosis iron is deposited in hepatocytes. In cirrhotic livers, parenchymal iron may be seen in patients with no other evidence of genetic haemochromatosis. Nevertheless the presence of any hepatocyte iron raises the possibility of genetic haemochromatosis, which must be excluded by appropriate iron studies. This pattern needs to be distinguished from haemosiderosis, in which iron is deposited in Kupffer cells. There are a number of causes for the latter appearance but in patients with hepatitis C the most common is treatment with ribavirin, which induces a haemolytic anaemia, and blood transfusion. In Egyptian patients, schistosome eggs may be identified within the portal tracts.

Sometimes in patients with hepatitis C, the liver biopsy may also provide a clue as to the means whereby the hepatitis C virus was contracted. For example, the presence of refractile foreign material, including talc particles, in the portal tracts is typically seen in patients who are past or present intravenous drug users. Examining sections under polarized light is helpful in identifying these particles.

Grading and staging of chronic viral hepatitis

The grading and staging of chronic viral hepatitis, and especially hepatitis C, has become a common, albeit much debated, undertaking. One of the most important

Figure 2.12
Liver from a patient with
HCV who also has brown
pigment in periportal
hepatocytes.

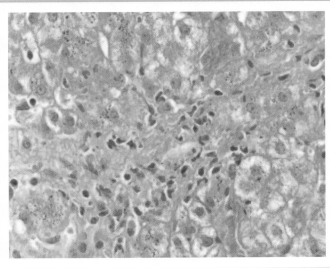

Figure 2.13
The same liver biopsy as
in 2.12 stained
specifically for iron (Perls
stain). The presence of
parenchymal iron is
strongly suggestive of
genetic
haemochromatosis.

recent conceptual developments in liver pathology has been the realization that when assessing liver biopsies from patients with chronic hepatitis it is essential to make a separate assessment of the severity of the necroinflammatory changes and the fibrotic changes. These two types of change are described by:

- the grade (for the necroinflammatory changes); and
- the stage (for fibrosis) respectively.

Grade essentially summarizes the overall severity of the inflammatory changes (Figs 2.8–2.11, 2.14) that are seen in and around the portal tracts and within the lobules, while stage provides information as to how far down the road to cirrhosis the patient has travelled (Figs 2.15–2.17). These terms were coined by analogy with the grading and staging of cancers. The grade depends on host and viral factors as well as on the effects of treatment, and it may wax and wane, especially in hepatitis C. On the other hand, until recently (and still controversially), fibrosis (measured by stage) was thought to be an irreversible process (see page 127). It should, nevertheless, be made clear that inflammation and fibrosis are related to each other pathophysiologically.

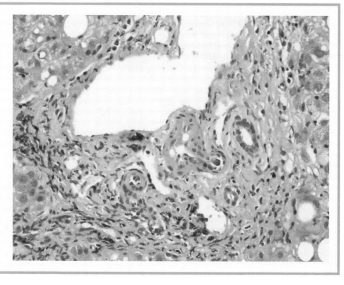

Figure 2.14
Liver biopsy showing a normal portal tract with scanty lymphocytes.

Figure 2.15
Liver biopsy showing a normal portal tract (Reticulin stain). On any of the scoring systems described this is Stage 0 disease.

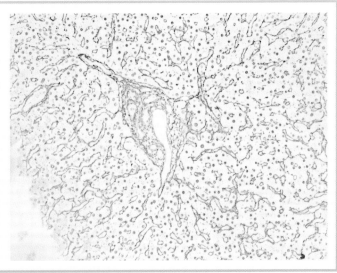

Figure 2.16
Liver biopsy showing bridging fibrosis with a portal tract connected to a central vein by connective tissue (Reticulin stain).

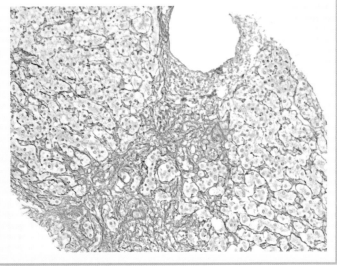

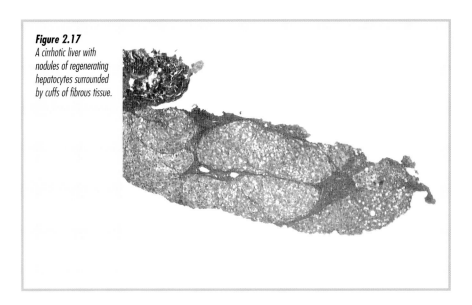

Figure 2.17
A cirrhotic liver with nodules of regenerating hepatocytes surrounded by cuffs of fibrous tissue.

While the definitions of portal and lobular inflammation are straightforward; the definition of interface hepatitis is less so. It is defined by two features:

- portal inflammation crossing the limiting plate (which is the line that separates the connective tissue of the portal tract from the hepatocytes) and extending into the lobules; and
- the presence of degenerative changes in the periportal hepatocytes.

The second feature distinguishes interface hepatitis from simple 'spill-over' of portal tract inflammation into the lobules, although in practice this distinction is very difficult. The term 'piecemeal necrosis' was coined to describe this progressive nibbling away of hepatocytes adjacent to the limiting plate. Purists object to the term 'piecemeal necrosis' because the mode of cell death seen is in fact apoptosis and not necrosis. For this reason the terms 'interface hepatitis' or 'periportal inflammation' have been suggested as being more accurate terms and the former is used here. However, as is so often the case when it comes to medical terminology, the use of the older term is likely to continue for some time to come. It is important to note that interface hepatitis can be seen not only in chronic hepatitis, of any cause, but also in other diseases such as primary biliary cirrhosis and Wilson's disease.

A number of different semiquantitative scoring systems have been proposed for assessing the grade and stage of the histopathological changes seen in chronic hepatitis C. They can be (and have been) applied to other causes of chronic hepatitis but they have been studied in most detail with reference to hepatitis C and are therefore discussed here. The four most widely used (Table 2.3) are:

- the histological activity index (HAI) or Knodell scoring system;
- the Scheuer scoring system;
- the METAVIR scoring system; and
- the modified HAI (Ishak) scoring system.

The Knodell (HAI) scoring system

The Knodell scoring system is the oldest liver biopsy scoring system. In its original form the scores for portal, periportal and lobular inflammation were added to the fibrosis score to give an overall HAI. After the importance of separating the necroinflammatory (grade) and fibrosis (stage) scores was appreciated (see page 35), this system has been modified. The scores for the inflammatory components have been split off; when added together they give the Knodell HAI inflammation score. The fibrosis gives the Knodell HAI fibrosis score.

Table 2.3
Summary of the four main biopsy scoring systems for chronic hepatitis

Scoring system	Maximum stage score	Maximum grade score	Comments
HAI (Knodell)	6	18	The original scoring system, which has been modified to separate stage and grade
Scheuer	4	4	The first scoring system to separate stage and grade
METAVIR	4	4	An excellent scoring system
Modified HAI (Ishak)	6	18	The most widely used scoring system in the UK and the USA

An idiosyncrasy of the Knodell scoring system is that the scores for the individual components are 0, 1, 3 and 4 (i.e. there is no 2). The reason for this is not clear but it does have the effect of separating scores into low-score groups (0 and 1) and high-score groups (3 and 4) with no intermediate groups. This feature is, however, an ongoing source of frustration to statisticians analysing studies in which this scoring system has been used.

Despite this drawback, the Knodell scoring system remains the one most widely used in clinical trials. It is a robust system that has been used for some time.

The Scheuer scoring system

Although not widely used except in Australia, the importance of the classic paper in which the Scheuer scoring system was described is that it was the first paper in which the importance of separating inflammatory and fibrosis scores was clearly stated and the first paper to use the terms 'grade' and 'stage' in this context.

The METAVIR scoring system

The METAVIR scoring system is an excellent scoring system that was developed by a group of French pathologists. It is the best validated of all the scoring systems in terms of its reproducibility and clinical application. The overall necroinflammatory score is read off a grid that has the score for interface hepatitis along one axis and the score for lobular inflammation along the other. The degree of portal inflammation is ignored because it is considered to be less important than interface hepatitis and lobular inflammation in producing liver damage. Unfortunately this system has not been widely used outside France.

The Ishak (modified HAI) scoring system

The Ishak scoring system (Table 2.4) is essentially an update of the Knodell (HAI) scoring system – grade and stage are clearly separated and there is no missing number in the scores for each feature (e.g. the scores for fibrosis go 0, 1, 2, 3, 4, 5, 6).

In addition there is a separate scoring category for confluent necrosis. It should be noted that confluent necrosis is in fact very unusual in chronic hepatitis C virus infection.

Another modification is that there are more points on each scale. For example, in the Knodell scoring system, there are four possible scores for fibrosis whereas in the Ishak scoring system there are seven. Although this increased sensitivity may appear an advantage it is not clear that

Table 2.4
The Ishak (modified HAI) scoring system

A.   Necroinflammatory score (grade)
Features to be scored
1.   Interface hepatitis (maximum possible score, 4)
2.   Confluent necrosis (maximum possible score, 6)
3.   Lobular inflammation (maximum possible score, 4)
4.   Portal inflammation (maximum possible score, 4)

1 + 2 +3 + 4 = necroinflammatory score (maximum possible score, 18)

B.   Fibrosis (stage)
Normal liver architecture (score, 0) to cirrhosis (maximum possible score, 6)

---

this feature is of benefit either in clinical practice or in trials. The reproducibility of this scoring system has been shown to be less than for the three other main scoring systems.

Overall comments

All the scoring systems described above have much in common. In all of them the scores for the individual histological features are ordinal data – that is, the scores increase with increasing severity of pathology – but the differences between the individual scores are not equal (and in fact are not known). For example, in the Ishak scoring system 0 means no fibrosis, 1 means focal portal tract expansion, while 2 means generalized portal tract expansion and 3 means focal bridging fibrosis. However, the significance of a

change of a score from 0 to 1 is unlikely to be the same as the significance of a score from 2 to 3 – the latter change is likely to be more clinically significant because bridging fibrosis is more likely to lead to cirrhosis.

All of the scores generated by any of the scoring systems are, by definition, non-parametric and therefore the appropriate statistical tests need to be applied when analysing them. A reading of the literature will reveal that this has not always been the case!

The question of inter- and intraobserver variation has been examined. The overall conclusion is that for experienced liver pathologists there is reasonably good inter- and intraobserver agreement.

Furthermore, the level of agreement is better for fibrosis scores than for inflammation scores.

A liver biopsy takes a sample of an extremely small fraction of the liver's mass. There is also, therefore, a question of sampling error. This has not been as carefully examined as interobserver variation but it does appear that it is a significant problem, especially in hepatitis C, which tends to show more focal changes than hepatitis B. To minimize the effect of sampling error it is important that a liver biopsy should be of adequate size before it can be assessed. Although there are no hard data to support this assertion, it is generally accepted that a liver biopsy must have at least three portal tracts before it should be considered large enough. This correlates with a length of approximately 1.5 cm.

It should be remembered that these scoring systems were designed for use in clinical trials, in which the use of a sufficiently large number of biopsies minimizes the impact of these two sources of error. Care must be taken when comparing the scores of just two different biopsies from the same patient, in which the significance of small differences should not be overestimated.

To score or not to score

Just because liver biopsies can be scored does not mean that it is always necessary to do so. In the setting of clinical trials where change in histology is one of the end-points it is clearly important to quantify the histological appearance, and the scoring systems were originally designed for this purpose. In routine clinical practice liver biopsy scores may be helpful to those centres that use the scores to determine clinical management but many centres prefer to assess liver biopsies from patients with chronic hepatitis C simply as 'mild', 'moderate' or 'severe' and there is no evidence that this approach is less valuable than formal scoring. Personal preference is probably the most important determinant of whether or not scoring should be used. There is certainly no point in the histopathologist scoring biopsies if the clinician is not going to act on this information.

The role of liver biopsy in the management of chronic hepatitis C

The major role of the liver biopsy in the management of chronic hepatitis C is twofold (Tables 2.5 and 2.6):

Table 2.5
Indications for liver biopsy in chronic hepatitis

To assess grade and stage
To assess response to treatment
To exclude coexisting causes of liver disease (e.g. haemochromatosis, hepatitis delta virus infection)
To assess dysplasia and malignancy

Table 2.6
A typical liver biopsy report from a patient with HCV

Macro
A core of brown tissue 3.1 cm
Micro
Liver with expansion of portal tracts with focal bridging fibrosis. There is moderate portal tract inflammation with poorly formed lymphoid aggregates. Hepatitic bile duct damage is seen, but there is no bile duct loss. There is mild interface hepatitis and moderate lobular inflammation. The latter is associated with moderate large droplet fatty change, but there is no fatty liver hepatitis. Special stains for iron, alpha-1 anti-trypsin bodies and copper-associated protein are negative. There is no dysplasia.
Conclusion
A moderate chronic hepatitis with features consistent with HCV.
Modified HAI score
Grade – 1+0+2+2=5/18
Stage – 3/6

- to determine whether any other disease process is present and to exclude significant iron overload, which may be exacerbated by ribavirin therapy; and
- to determine the severity of the liver disease in order to facilitate the decision as to whether or not therapy should be given and to act as a baseline for assessing subsequent disease progression.

The role of liver biopsy management is discussed in more detail in Chapter 3.

Further reading

Bartenschlager R, Lohmann V. Replication of hepatitis C virus. *J Gen Virol* 2000; **81:** 1631–48.

Brunt EM. Grading and staging the histopathological lesions of chronic hepatitis: the Knodell histology activity index and beyond. *Hepatology* 2000; **31:** 241–6.

Hall PD. Broadsheet number 47. Chronic hepatitis: an update with guidelines for histopathological assessment of liver biopsies. Board of Education of The Royal College of Pathologists of Australasia. *Pathology* 1998; **30:** 369–80.

Lefkowitch JH, Schiff ER, Davis GL, *et al.* Pathological diagnosis of chronic hepatitis C: a multicenter comparative study with chronic hepatitis B. The Hepatitis Interventional Therapy Group. *Gastroenterology* 1993; **104:** 595–603.

Poynard T, Bedossa P, Opolon P. Natural history of liver fibrosis progression in patients with chronic hepatitis C. *Lancet* 1997; **349:** 825–32.

Saadeh S, Cammell G, Carey WD, Younossi Z, Barnes D, Easley K. The role of liver biopsy in chronic hepatitis C. *Hepatology* 2001; **33:** 196–200.

Scheuer PJ, Ashrafzadeh P, Sherlock S, *et al.* The pathology of hepatitis C. *Hepatology* 1992; **15:** 567–71.

Simmonds P, Holmes EC, Cha TA, *et al.* Classification of hepatitis C virus into six major genotypes and a series of subtypes by phylogenetic analysis of the NS-5 region. *J Gen Virol* 1993; **74:** 2391–9.

Questions

1. In chronic hepatitis C virus infection:
   A. Different genotypes cause disease that progresses at a different rate
   B. Patients infected with genotype 1 require 48 weeks of therapy
   C. Genotype 4 is common in western Europe
   D. Genotype is commonly determined by examining the sequence of the 5′ non-coding region
   E. The viral genotype can be used to predict the likelihood of cirrhosis

2. In chronic hepatitis C virus infection:
   A. Spontaneous clearance is common
   B. In general 30% of patients will develop cirrhosis after 30 years
   C. Alcohol consumption reduces the incidence of vascular disease and is likely to be beneficial

D. Patients with normal liver function tests do not need to undergo liver biopsy since mild disease is always found

E. Liver biopsy is the only reliable means of identifying the extent of the liver injury

3. In the assessment of a liver biopsy from a patient with chronic hepatitis C:
A. The grade of the biopsy indicates the amount of inflammation
B. A METAVIR stage 6 indicates cirrhosis
C. A modified HAI (Ishak) stage of 4 indicates cirrhosis
D. The presence of fat confirms alcohol abuse
E. Granulomas are common

4. In a patient with chronic hepatitis C:
A. Excess iron deposition in the liver is common and should be ignored
B. Lymphoid aggregates are common
C. Age less than 40 at the time of infection may accelerate the progression of the disease
D. A fibrosis score of 4 indicates that the disease is twice as severe as a score of 3
E. Dactopenia is common

Answers

Question 1

A. False
B. True
C. False
D. True
E. False

Question 2

A. False
B. True
C. False – alcohol use accelerates the progression of the liver disease and should always be discouraged
D. False – a proportion of patients with normal liver function tests have severe disease
E. True

Question 3

A. True
B. False – stage 4 in the METAVIR system indicates cirrhosis
C. False – stage 6 in the modified HAI (Ishak scoring system) indicates cirrhosis
D. False – fat is common in patients with hepatitis C
E. False

Question 4

A. False – excess iron deposition requires investigation and possibly therapy

B. True

C. False – patients infected when they are young tend to have less aggressive disease

D. False – the fibrosis scales are non-linear

E. False

Diagnosis and management of chronic hepatitis C virus infection

3

Patients with chronic hepatitis C virus infection are referred for therapy from a wide variety of health-care workers. For all patients who are infected with hepatitis C virus, it is important to confirm the diagnosis and assess the severity of the disease before planning therapy.

Diagnosis of chronic HCV

Patients who are suspected of having chronic hepatitis C virus infection are normally tested for exposure to the virus with an assay that detects antibodies against the virus. A number of different assays are commercially available; some (such as the enzyme immunoassay EIA) detect whether antibodies are present or absent while others (such as the RIBA assays) identify the antibody target proteins in more detail. (RIBA assays usually provide information on the binding of antibodies to four or five antigens from hepatitis C virus. If two or more are positive, the test indicates exposure to hepatitis C. A single positive is regarded as indeterminate.)

Both types of assay, when positive, confirm that the patient has been exposed to the hepatitis C virus. With most viruses, the presence of circulating antibodies indicates past, resolved infection with that virus rather than ongoing infection. This is not the case with the hepatitis C virus – antibodies against the hepatitis C virus are found in patients who are actively infected.

> All patients who have antibodies against hepatitis C virus must be investigated in detail to determine whether they have eliminated the virus or whether they are still infected.

> The diagnosis of chronic hepatitis C rests on detection of the virus in blood by a sensitive nucleic acid detection assay (e.g. a polymerase chain reaction [PCR] assay) to detect viral RNA.

Liver function tests should be measured in all patients suspected of having hepatitis C but normal liver function tests do not exclude infection since many infected patients have transiently or persistently normal liver function tests. Equally, the presence of antibodies against hepatitis C virus and abnormal liver function tests does not confirm the diagnosis of chronic hepatitis C virus infection, since another cause for the liver abnormalities may be present. Hence, all patients who have

detectable antibodies against the hepatitis C virus should have a sample of serum analysed for the presence of virus by a sensitive assay (usually a PCR assay) that is capable of detecting 50 iu/ml (50 iu of virus is equivalent to 100 copies).

A small proportion of patients have detectable antibodies but are persistently 'PCR-negative' – they have undetectable viraemia. In our practice this is rare and less than 5% of our patients present in this way. Such patients have presumably been exposed to hepatitis C virus but have eliminated the virus spontaneously. Once this diagnosis has been confirmed no further follow-up is required, but it is important to test the hepatitis C PCR on three separate occasions since low-level, fluctuating viraemia may confound the diagnosis.

Occasionally, patients are seen who do not have detectable antibodies against hepatitis C virus but who are viraemic (i.e. they have detectable hepatitis C virus RNA). This may be seen in patients who are heavily immunosuppressed or who have contracted the infection within the previous few weeks (the antibody response typically takes a few months to develop and hence early infection may be characterized by viraemia in the absence of antibodies). In these patients, a high index of suspicion is required to identify the infection correctly.

Following confirmation of the diagnosis it is important to counsel the patient about infectivity and the effects of the infection on partners and other family members. The issues about transmission of the hepatitis C virus are described in detail in Chapter 1, and the natural history of the infection is discussed in Chapter 2. Table 3.1 summarizes the important issues that should be discussed with all infected patients at the time of diagnosis.

Once the diagnosis of chronic hepatitis C virus infection has been established, a liver biopsy should be performed to grade and stage the disease (see page 35). At this juncture it is helpful to identify confounding diseases that may complicate therapy. The investigations that should be performed before therapy is started are listed in Table 3.2.

Therapy of chronic hepatitis C virus infection

Treatment of chronic hepatitis C virus infection is based around interferon-alpha

Table 3.1
Issues to be discussed when counseling a patient with newly diagnosed chronic HCV

Issue		Comment
Natural history		Typically slow – only 30% of patients develop cirrhosis after 30 years
Organ/blood donation		Infected patients must not donate
Transmission	Sex	Risk of sexual transmission is low, less than 3%
	Close contact	Transmission risk is nil
	Household contact	Very low risk but do not share blood stained items (e.g. toothbrush, razor etc)
	Mother-baby	Transmission risk is less than 5%
	Breast feeding	Transmission risk is nil
	Sharing needles and injecting paraphenalia	High risk of transmission – must be avoided
Alcohol		Excess alcohol increases the rate of liver damage and even moderate/light drinking may be harmful
Therapy		Combination therapy may cure over 50% of infected patients

Table 3.2
Investigations that should be performed prior to starting therapy for patients with chronic hepatitis C infection

Investigation		Comment
Hepatitis C RNA PCR		Confirms the diagnosis. Some groups assess the level of viraemia (quantitative PCR) and use the level to modify the duration of therapy
Hepatitis B serology		If co-infection with hepatitis B is confirmed consider alternative treatment approaches
HIV		Should be considered in all patients and, if the patient is regarded as high risk testing for HIV co-infection should be performed after appropriate consent.
Liver function tests		Important baseline investigation
Renal function		Impaired renal function may require dose of ribavirin to be adjusted
Full blood count	Haemoglobin	Likely to fall by 2–3 gm during therapy
	White cell count	Will decrease during therapy
	Platelet count	Will decrease during therapy
Thyroid function tests		May deteriorate during therapy
Serum ferritin		If markedly raised (>3 times the upper limit normal) indicates iron overload which may impair the response to therapy
Autoantibodies		If present at a titre > 1:80 re-consider the diagnosis
Pregnancy test		Ribavirin is contraindicated in pregnant women
ECG		For patients at risk of significant heart disease
Chest X ray		For patients at risk of significant heart and lung disease

derivatives. All of these drugs are given by repeated subcutaneous injection for many months and are associated with a wide range of side effects, including:

- fever;
- fatigue;
- nausea;
- depression;
- hair loss.

The natural history of chronic hepatitis C virus infection is highly variable (see page 25). In some patients the disease progresses very slowly, and infirmity and death develop long before significant liver damage occurs; however, in others the disease follows a more rapid course, and death from cirrhosis or liver cancer occurs in middle age. For those patients who have non-progressive disease, the side effects of therapy are likely to be worse than the consequences of the disease, and therefore therapy should be reserved for those patients who are likely to develop significant problems as a result of their infection.

Selection of patients for treatment

> *The main goal of patient selection is to identify those patients who have, or who are likely to develop, significant liver damage.*

> *It is impossible to identify the degree of liver damage from liver function tests and therefore adequate pretreatment assessment requires a liver biopsy.*

The liver biopsy allows an accurate assessment of liver injury and permits confirmation that the liver disease is due entirely to hepatitis C. In general, patients with mild liver damage should not be treated, and therapy should be reserved for those with moderate to severe disease. The precise definition of moderate to

severe disease is necessarily dependent on individual circumstances – for example, in a 65-year-old man with ischaemic heart disease the degree of liver damage required to justify therapy is greater than that required in an otherwise healthy 25-year-old patient. Most liver units agree to treat patients whose degree of fibrosis exceeds a pre-set limit or who have significant inflammation.

Selection based on liver histology

To ensure equity of access to therapy for hepatitis C and to ensure that all patients are treated appropriately, most liver centres have established severity criteria that must be met before a patient is eligible for treatment. Different groups have established slightly different criteria and it is unlikely that the different regimes will be compared in any formal studies. Our policy is to score all liver biopsies using the modified histological activity index (modified HAI [Ishak]) scoring system, and patients are eligible for treatment if they have a fibrosis score of greater than 2. Since patients with minimal fibrosis who have marked necroinflammation may be at greater risk of developing progressive disease, we also offer therapy to all patients who have a total necroinflammatory score of greater than 3.

It is important to recognize that the

development of liver fibrosis in patients with chronic hepatitis C may not be linear and that past fibrosis may be a poor indicator of future damage. Patients who have not been treated because their biopsy indicates that the disease is mild should be reviewed on a regular basis and should have a repeat liver biopsy after 3–5 years. If the repeat biopsy shows evidence of progressive fibrosis we would recommend therapy at that stage, but if the biopsy shows no evidence of disease progression follow-up without therapy is appropriate. Since sampling error can lead to small changes in the histological scores, we regard progressive disease as a change of more than 1 in the fibrosis score.

Other indications for therapy

Many patients with chronic hepatitis C complain of a variety of non-specific symptoms, chiefly fatigue, upper abdominal pain, difficulty in concentrating and joint pain (see page 115). These symptoms are independent of the degree of liver damage and they often improve with successful therapy. In patients who are severely disabled by their associated symptoms it is reasonable to offer therapy even if the liver damage is mild. Many patients with chronic hepatitis C have a past history of intravenous drug abuse and a high proportion have a past history of psychiatric disorders, typically requiring outpatient therapy. In patients with psychiatric symptoms eradication of the virus does not improve quality of life, and it is important not to raise expectations in those with a past history of minor mental illness.

Alternative approaches to biopsy-based management algorithms

At present, therapy for chronic hepatitis C virus infection is based on liver histology, and treatment is reserved for those with active disease. This approach has been endorsed by both North American and European consensus conferences and is based on therapies that are in current use (standard interferon plus ribavirin). The rationale behind the development of biopsy-based algorithms is that therapy for hepatitis C is poorly effective, poorly tolerated and expensive. If a potent, inexpensive treatment that was free of side effects were developed, it is likely that all patients with hepatitis C would be treated, regardless of the extent of the liver damage, and the inconvenience, costs and risks involved in assessment of disease activity by liver biopsy would therefore be avoided.

New, long-acting, pegylated interferons (i.e. interferons linked to a polyethylene glycol – see page 56) are currently being assessed. It is not yet clear whether these modified interferons will be sufficiently effective, tolerable and cheap to justify a change from biopsy-based treatment algorithms. The sustained response rates for patients with hepatitis C of genotypes 2 and 3 approach 80% with pegylated interferon plus ribavirin therapy, and the combination is well tolerated. It is therefore likely that a change in current practice will be discussed over the next few years. The costs of the new pegylated interferons may determine whether all patients with hepatitis C of genotypes 2 and 3 receive therapy or whether therapy remains restricted to those with active disease.

For patients with hepatitis C of genotype 1, response rates with the new pegylated interferons remain suboptimal and it is likely that biopsy-based management algorithms will remain in use for the foreseeable future in these patients.

Defining 'cure' – lessons from past errors

The early clinical trials for chronic hepatitis C virus infection used interferon-alpha monotherapy and led to enthusiastic reports of 'cure' rates approaching 50%. Unfortunately these early trials defined a cure as 'normal liver function tests at the end of therapy', and it soon became clear that many patients with normal liver function tests at the end

of therapy go on to relapse during follow-up. Later studies analysed the response to treatment by measuring viral RNA at the end of therapy, and such studies showed that some patients with normal liver function tests remain viraemic, a situation that leads to further distortion of the sustained response rates. Hence early clinical trials used inappropriate end-points and grossly overestimated the proportion of patients who were cured.

The lessons from these early treatment trials have led to the adoption of strict criteria for treatment response.

> A 'sustained response' to therapy is now defined as normalization of liver function tests and undetectable hepatitis C viral RNA (by a sensitive molecular assay) 6 months after cessation of therapy.

If this strict definition is used, then patients who show a sustained response to therapy have a greater than 95% chance of remaining non-viraemic with normal liver biochemistry and improved hepatic histology 10 years after the end of therapy. To all intents and purposes these patients are cured. Purists may argue that cure can only be determined when patients have died of a cause that is unrelated to hepatitis C. Occasional relapses many years after therapy do occur (although they are very rare, probably occurring in less than 1% of patients) and therefore annual follow-up of all treatment responders may be prudent.

For patients who have been cured there is often debate as to whether immunosuppression will lead to viral recurrence (as does occur with hepatitis B virus infection). There are no data to suggest that immunosuppression may lead to relapse but it would seem wise to continue to monitor these patients until more is known about the long-term outcome.

Treatment options in chronic hepatitis C

> For patients with chronic hepatitis C virus infection the optimum therapy is combination therapy with an interferon and ribavirin.

Ribavirin is a modified nucleoside analogue that has antiviral activity against a wide range of different viruses. In addition to its antiviral effects, ribavirin can activate Th1 cells and thereby facilitate immunological clearance of an infecting virus (see page 6).

When used as monotherapy for patients with chronic hepatitis C virus infection, ribavirin is disappointing and has no demonstrable antiviral effects, although it may improve the liver function tests by an unidentified mechanism. When ribavirin is combined with interferon in the therapy of chronic hepatitis C, the two drugs are synergistic and the combination is markedly more effective than either drug given alone.

The mechanism of action of ribavirin in this setting is unclear and it is not known whether the synergistic effects seen with interferon and ribavirin are due to the antiviral activity of ribavirin or to its immunomodulatory properties.

Although ribavirin increases the efficacy of interferon therapy it also increases the side effects. Ribavirin induces mild haemolysis that leads to a reduction in the haemoglobin concentration of 2–3 g/dl. This mild anaemia tends to exacerbate the interferon-related malaise, and many patients receiving combination therapy become profoundly fatigued. Recent reports suggest that therapy with erythropoetin may increase the haemoglobin level in patients receiving ribavirin, but whether this improves compliance and is cost effective has not yet been determined. Ribavirin may induce nausea, a chronic cough and small oral ulcers, and it occasionally causes troublesome dry, scaly skin lesions.

Although most patients tolerate these side effects, for some the therapy is intolerable and ribavirin has to be discontinued.

Choice of interferon

The type I interferons are a family of natural cytokines that are produced as part of the innate immune response against viral infections (see page 3). The interferon proteins have been isolated and the genes that encode them have been cloned, so that a variety of type I interferons are now commercially available. They are widely used in the therapy of viral infections as well as in the treatment of some malignant tumours. A number of unmodified, 'standard' interferons are available, including:

- recombinant naturally occurring interferons (interferon-alpha-2a – Roferon – and interferon-alpha-2b – Intron); and
- recombinant, modified interferon (consensus interferon – Infergen).
- natural interferons (e.g. Alferon, Sumiferon), which are derived from viral infection of leukocytes or lymphocytes;

All of these interferons are of similar potency – when used at a dose of 3–6 Miu three times a week for 48 weeks, 10–20% of patients will be cured by standard interferon monotherapy. Increasing the dose of these interferons beyond 6 Miu three times a week adds little to their efficacy and is not recommended.

All of the currently available 'standard' interferons have a very short half-life and have to be given at least three times a week by subcutaneous injection. Increasing the half-life of these interferons by linking them to a polyethylene glycol moiety increases their clinical efficacy, and the pegylated interferons are rapidly becoming the treatment of choice for patients with chronic hepatitis C virus infection. The pegylated interferons are injected once a week and, although their side effect profile is similar to the standard interferons, the side effects are less marked and the drugs are better tolerated than the parent interferons. Two pegylated interferons are currently available; the differences between them are summarized in Table 3.3.

Combination therapy – interferon and ribavirin

For patients with chronic hepatitis C virus infection, the combination of standard interferon with ribavirin leads to a sustained response rate of more than 40%.

Table 3.3
Comparison of the currently available pegylated interferons

	12 kD pegylated interferon-alpha-2b (Peg Intron)	40 kD pegylated interferon-alpha-2b (Pegasys)
Preparation	Dry powder – requires reconstitution with water before administration	Ready to inject liquid
Half life	40 ± 13.3 h	80 ± 32 h
Dose	1.5 µg/kg body weight (patients should be weighed and the dose of drug calculated according to body weight)	180 µg (standard dose for all patients regardless of body weight)
Efficacy as monotherapy	23–25% of patients are cured	30–39% of patients are cured
Efficacy when combined with ribavirin	54% cure*	56% cure[†]

Trials to-date have combined 1.5 µg/kg of 12 kD pegylated interferon-alpha-2b with 800 mg/day of ribavirin. It is not yet clear whether increasing the dose of ribavirin increases the response rates.
[†] *Trials to date have combined 40 kD pegylated interferon-alpha-2a with 1000 mg or 1200 mg of ribavirin. Trials to determine whether lower doses of ribavirin are equally effective are currently in progress.*

It is important to use an adequate dose of ribavirin since decreasing the dose below an appropriate level decreases the response rate. Ribavirin dosing is dependent on the weight of the patient – 1000 mg should be used in patients weighing less than 75 kg; 1200 mg is the correct dose for those weighing more than this.

The appropriate duration of combination therapy with standard interferon and ribavirin depends on the genotype of the infecting virus. For patients infected with hepatitis C virus of genotype 1, therapy for 48 weeks (virtually 12 months) is needed, but for those infected with genotypes 2 or 3, treatment is required for no more than 24 weeks (virtually 6 months). The correct duration of treatment for patients infected with multiple genotypes or with other genotypes is not clear, but we routinely use 48 weeks' therapy for all patients other than those infected with genotypes 2 or 3. Patients with hepatitis C of genotype 1 who have a low viral load (defined as less than 2×10^6 viral copies/ml – equivalent to 800,000 iu/ml) may require only 6 months of therapy, but this is controversial. Patients with hepatitis C of genotype 1 who have not responded after 6 months treatment should have therapy withdrawn because a response is very unlikely (i.e. patients infected with hepatitis C virus of genotype 1 who remain viraemic – virus detectable in blood – after 24 weeks of combination therapy should discontinue treatment). Figure 3.1 outlines the management of patients receiving therapy with interferon and ribavirin.

The long-acting pegylated interferons have been assessed in combination with ribavirin and they appear to be significantly more effective than standard interferon plus ribovirin, with sustained response rates of greater than 50%.

The appropriate duration of therapy with the new pegylated interferons and

ribavirin is not yet known. Clinical trials to date have used 48 weeks of therapy in all patients, including those with genotypes 2 and 3. It is likely that patients with 'easy to treat genotypes' will require only 24 weeks of therapy with the pegylated interferons and ribavirin, but this has not yet been formally proven.

The dose of ribavirin that is required with these new interferons is also under review. Clinical trials with the 12 kD pegylated interferon-alpha-2b have used a fixed ribavirin dose of 800 mg. It is not known whether increasing the dose of ribavirin will increase the response rates or whether the higher doses will lead to more side effects and more treatment failures. For the well-tolerated 40 kD pegylated interferon-alpha-2a, clinical trials have used standard doses (1000 mg or 1200 mg) of ribavirin, and trials with lower doses are currently under way.

The effectiveness of combination therapy with the 40 kD pegylated interferon-alpha-2a can be assessed after only 3 months of therapy. If the patient has not lost virus after 12 weeks of therapy (i.e. hepatitis C virus testing shows that the virus is still present) or if the level of circulating viraemia (assessed by quantitative testing) has not fallen by at least 100-fold (a 2 log drop) then the patient has a very low

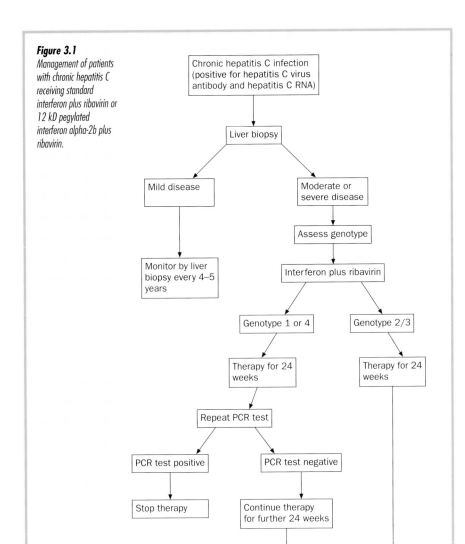

Figure 3.1
Management of patients with chronic hepatitis C receiving standard interferon plus ribavirin or 12 kD pegylated interferon alpha-2b plus ribavirin.

probability (less than 3%) of responding to therapy. Hence unsuccessful therapy with the 40 kD pegylated interferon-alpha-2a and ribavirin can be discontinued after only 3 months, sparing patients the side effects of prolonged therapy. It is not yet known whether the response to the 12 kD pegylated interferon-alpha-2b can be predicted in this way.

Figure 3.2 shows a clinical algorithm for the management of patients with the new 40 kD pegylated interferon plus ribavirin.

Management during interferon and ribavirin therapy
Pretreatment assessment

> *Ribavirin is teratogenic in animals and it is very likely that conception while receiving ribavirin will lead to fetal abnormalities.*

It is essential that all fertile women planning to start ribavirin should be screened for pregnancy before therapy and all should be taking adequate contraceptive precautions. Past experience convinces us that 'careful abstinence' in single women is not an effective contraceptive and we insist that all women of child-bearing age take regular contraceptives or carry condoms

at all times. Since ribavirin has a long half-life, effective contraception should be continued for at least 6 months after therapy.

> *Animal studies suggest that ribavirin can cause defects in sperm, leading males to father deformed offspring.*

It is important that all men planning to commence therapy take effective contraceptive precautions for the duration of therapy and for a further 6 months after therapy.

All patients should be carefully assessed before starting combination therapy. The full blood count should be reviewed and patients who are anaemic (haemoglobin less than 11 g/dl), thrombocytopenic (platelet count less than 70×10^9 cells/l) or neutropenic (neutrophil count less than 1×10^9 cells/l) should not normally be commenced on combination therapy. In patients over the age of 40, a chest X-ray and ECG is prudent to exclude significant pulmonary and cardiac disease that may be exacerbated by ribavirin-associated anaemia. The hepatological investigations should always be reviewed before therapy to confirm the diagnosis, and thyroid function should be evaluated.

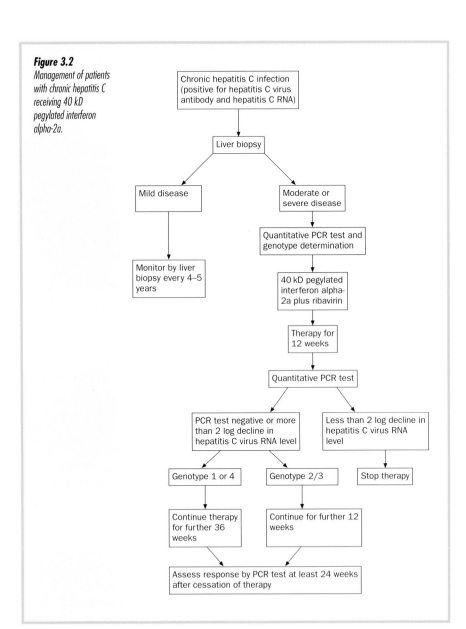

Figure 3.2
Management of patients with chronic hepatitis C receiving 40 kD pegylated interferon alpha-2a.

One of the most feared complications of interferon therapy is suicidal depression, probably related to an interferon-induced reduction in serotonin levels in the central nervous system.

> *Severe depression caused by interferon is rare but when it does occur it may progress rapidly and lead to attempted suicide.*

Characteristically the patient becomes profoundly depressed and loses insight such that the cause of the depression (interferon therapy) is not apparent. All patients receiving interferon should be assessed before therapy to determine the likelihood of severe depression. A past history of psychiatric disease requiring hospitalization may indicate an increased risk, and such patients should not normally receive interferon therapy. Patients who have received outpatient antidepressant therapy in the past may be treated with interferon but vigilance is required, and it may be wise to consider starting such patients on prophylactic antidepressant medication before starting therapy.

Management during therapy
Combination therapy with standard interferon and ribavirin is unpleasant.

After the first injection most patients complain of a fever, sweating, headaches and malaise. These flu-like symptoms tend to decrease in severity with each injection and can be improved by taking paracetamol 2 hours before the injection.

During the first few weeks of therapy ribavirin induces a haemolytic anaemia, and the hemoglobin typically falls by 2–3 g/dl. In some patients the decrease is greater than this and it becomes necessary to reduce the dose of ribavirin. A dose of less than 600 mg is probably not effective, and if such a reduction is needed, the drug should be discontinued and interferon monotherapy (preferably with one of the pegylated forms) used instead.

The leukocyte and platelet count decline during the first few weeks of therapy as a result of interferon-induced myelosuppression, and this may necessitate a reduction in the dose of interferon – usually to 2 Miu thrice weekly. For the 40 kD pegylated interferon, the dose should be reduced to 135 mg for a few weeks in patients who have developed neutropenia or thrombocytopenia, but if the full blood count improves on a reduced dose then it is often possible to return to the full dose without further problems. Similar approaches have been used with the 12 kD pegylated interferon.

Hair loss typically develops after 3 months of therapy and is associated with hair thinning. Patients should be reassured that the hair will grow again but that full recovery will take many months after treatment has stopped.

Impotence is common; it is reversible on stopping therapy and most patients are satisfied with reassurance.

Thyorid dysfunction is common in those with a family history of thyroid disease, but it can also occur in patients with no predisposing factors. We routinely measure thyroid function tests every 3 months while patients are receiving treatment, and both hypothyroidism and hyperthyroidism may be found. Fortunately, this complication, which is often permanent, responds well to standard therapy.

The side effect profile of the pegylated interferons appears to be similar to that seen with the unmodified interferons, although the severity of the flu-like symptoms may be diminished. Changes in haematological parameters may be more marked with the pegylated interferons, and these should be carefully monitored throughout therapy.

Common side effects and their management are listed in Table 3.4.

Difficult-to-treat patients
Active drug users

Most patients with chronic hepatitis C virus infection have a past history of injecting drug use and some are actively using drugs when they are referred for therapy. Unfortunately patients who are actively using addictive drugs have been excluded from many of the current clinical trials and there are therefore no data about the safety and efficacy of therapy in this patient group. Some clinical trials have included patients who are receiving regular oral methadone, and there is no evidence of either impaired response rates or increased toxicity. Anecdotal reports suggest that patients who have recently withdrawn from methadone therapy may relapse when exposed to the rigors of combination therapy, and our policy is to treat patients who are receiving maintenance methadone rather than waiting for the patient to withdraw completely from opiates.

For patients who are actively using non-prescribed 'street' drugs there are unexplored risks relating to interactions with interferon and ribavirin. Clearly these patients are at greater risk of drug-related toxicity and they may have other, more pressing, health concerns. Current policy is therefore to defer treatment in patients who are using 'street' drugs, but

Table 3.4
Common side effects during combination therapy with interferon and ribavirin, and their management

Side effect	Management
Flu-like symptoms	Paracetamol to reduce severity of the symptoms
Cough	Cough linctus; the cough sometimes improves with a reduction in the dose of ribavirin
Dry, scaly skin rashes	May respond to local hydrocortisone cream (1%)
Hair loss	Reassurance
Mouth ulcers	Sugar-free gum to improve saliva flow
Anaemia	Reduce dose of ribavirin, but if a reduction to less than 600 mg is required it may be wise to withdraw the drug completely since low-dose ribavirin may not be effective
Neutropaenia	Reduce dose of interferon
Thrombocytopaenia	Reduce dose of interferon
Mild depression	Consider antidepressant medication
Psychoses	Stop therapy and arrange urgent psychiatric review
Thyroid dysfunction	Manage with standard regimes

each case should be assessed on its merits – therapy may be justified in compliant patients with advancing liver disease, and recent studies have shown that treatment in the patient group is safe and effective.

Associated liver autoantibodies

Chronic hepatitis C virus infection is occasionally associated with liver autoantibodies. In such patients the question arises as to whether the autoantibodies are coincidental or whether they are contributing to the liver damage. In some patients the histology provides a clue, but in many the dominant disease is not clear. Unusually large numbers of plasma cells and particularly active interface hepatitis suggest that autoimmune liver disease is the dominant problem (Figure 3.3), but the diagnosis is rarely clear-cut.

In these patients, therapy with prednisolone (for a presumed autoimmune disease) improves the liver function tests regardless of the underlying disease. However, if the primary cause of

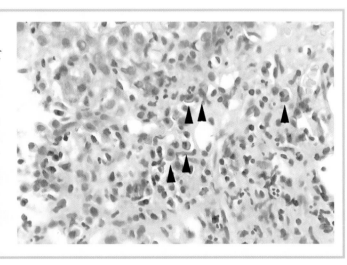

Figure 3.3
Liver biopsy from a patient with hepatitis C virus infection. The inflammatory infiltrate contains conspicuous plasma cells, which is unusual and raises the possibility of an autoimmune hepatitis.

the liver damage is infection with hepatitis C virus, the improvement in liver function tests may be associated with progression of the hepatic fibrosis. If these patients are treated with interferon and the main cause of the liver damage is immmuological, then the interferon induces a rapid deterioration in liver function tests – interferon withdrawal followed by immunosuppression is then the appropriate management option.

Hence, we recommend that these patients are commenced on interferon therapy to determine whether their primary hepatic disease is viral or immunological and, during this therapeutic trial, the liver function tests should be monitored closely. If the liver function tests improve, the liver disease is probably viral in origin, and antiviral therapy should be continued; if the serum transaminases increase, autoimmune disease is likely, and interferon should be withdrawn and therapy with prednisolone considered. These patients should be closely monitored by serial liver biopsies since progression of the fibrosis may occur.

Children
The natural history of chronic hepatitis C virus infection in children has not yet been defined – small-scale studies suggest that the disease is likely to be mild during

the first few years after infection but the long-term outlook is not clear and clearly the lifetime risk of liver complications must be considerable. Few clinical trials have been performed in children, and in view of the slow natural history in young people it is probably appropriate to treat children only in the context of controlled clinical trials.

Further reading

Foster G, Goldin R, Main J, Murray-Lyon I, Hargreaves S, Thomas H. The management of chronic hepatitis C: clinical audit of a biopsy based management algorithm. *BMJ* 1997; **315**: 453–8.

Marcellin P, Boyer N, Gervais A, *et al*. Long-term histologic improvement and loss of detectable intrahepatic HCV RNA in patients with chronic hepatitis C and sustained response to interferon-alpha therapy. *Ann Intern Med* 1997; **127**: 875–81.

Lauer GM, Walker BD. Hepatitis C infection. *N Engl J Med* 2001; **345**: 41–52.

McHutchison JG, Gordon SC, Schiff ER, *et al*. Interferon alfa-2b alone or in combination with ribavirin as initial treatment for chronic hepatitis C. Hepatitis Interventional Therapy Group. *N Engl J Med* 1998; **339**: 1485–92.

Moussalli J, Opolon P, Poynard T. Management of chronic hepatitis C. *J Viral Hep* 1998; **5**: 73–82.

Zeuzem S, Feinman SV, Rasenack J, *et al*. Peginterferon alfa-2a in patients with chronic hepatitis C. *N Engl J Med* 2000; **343**: 1666–72.

Questions

1. In the diagnosis of chronic hepatitis C virus infection:
   A. The presence of antibodies against the virus indicates past infection
   B. Normal liver function tests indicate that the virus has been eliminated
   C. A sensitive test that detects 50 iu/ml of hepatitis C virus RNA should be used in all patients
   D. Quantification of the hepatitis C virus RNA titre is not necessary to confirm the diagnosis
   E. Patient counselling increases patient anxiety and should be avoided

2. Ribavirin therapy for patients with chronic hepatitis C virus infection:
   A. Should be given by intramuscular injection
   B. Induces a haemolytic anaemia that may respond to therapy with erythropoietin

C. Is effective as monotherapy

D. Should not normally be used at doses of less than 600 mg

E. Synergizes with interferon by activating Th2 type responses.

3. Combination therapy with interferon and ribavirin in patients with chronic hepatitis C:
A. Is the treatment of choice
B. May cure over 50% of patients when a pegylated interferon is used
C. Can be used in pregnant women to reduce the risks of maternal–fetal transmission
D. May induce permanent thyroid disease
E. Requires regular assessment of white cell count and platelet count

4. Therapy for chronic hepatitis C virus infection:
A. Should be offered to patients with depression as viral clearance may improve fatigue-like symptoms
B. May require antidepressant therapy during treatment to reduce the drug related side effects
C. Is ineffective in patients with cirrhosis
D. Should be offered to patients with mild liver disease because response rates are higher in this group of patients

E. Should be avoided in patients with severe ischaemic heart disease

Answers

Question 1

A. False – in chronic hepatitis C virus infection antibodies coexist with the virus and hence the presence of antibodies usually indicates ongoing infection

B. False – liver function tests may be normal even in the presence of significant liver disease

C. True

D. True

E. False

Question 2

A. False – the drug should be used orally

B. True

C. False

D. True – in patients of average weight, doses less than 600 mg are probably ineffective

E. False. the drug synergizes by activating Th1 responses

Question 3

A. True

B. True

C. False – ribavirin is teratogenic and must be avoided in pregnant women
D. True
E. True

Question 4

A. False – interferon may aggravate pre-existing depression and carries a substantial risk of suicide in those with previous psychiatric disorders
B. True
C. False – response rates are reduced in patients with cirrhosis but a significant proportion of patients will respond
D. False
E. True

4

Hepatitis B – virology, natural history and pathology

The hepatitis B virus is an unusual virus – it is the smallest human pathogen and yet it causes more chronic infections than any other human virus. The hepatitis B viral genome was first sequenced in 1979 but the functions of some of the encoded proteins are still unclear. Like the hepatitis C virus and HIV, the hepatitis B virus mutates at a high rate and, as the disease progresses, new viral species develop that lead to different forms of the disease. Recent therapeutic developments involve nucleoside analogues that target the hepatitis B virus directly. These drugs significantly modify the course of chronic infection and may lead to the production of mutant viral strains with different characteristics.

Hepatitis B – the virus

Hepatitis B virus belongs to the Hepadnaviridae viral family. Other members of this group infect birds (such as Peking ducks and herons) as well as small rodents (such as woodchucks), and the availability of these small animal models of infection has greatly facilitated studies into the pathogenesis of the human form of hepatitis B virus infection. The virus is distantly related to the retroviruses that cause immunodeficiency syndromes, and the polymerase protein that duplicates the hepatitis B genome is sufficiently similar to the HIV polymerase for some drugs to inhibit both enzymes and act against both viruses.

Hepatitis B virus is a very small virus – the entire genome is only 3.2 kB long (i.e. the DNA that makes up the entire virus is smaller than some human genes). To compress all the information needed to produce an infectious agent into this very small genome, hepatitis B virus uses 'overlapping open reading frames' to encode the four proteins that make up the intact virus (Fig. 4.1). This overlapping genomic structure allows the hepatitis B virus to pack a large amount of genetic material into a very small genetic space. However, because many DNA bases code for more than one amino acid, many mutations are non-viable because they lead to the production of defective proteins. This is easily seen by examining the overlap between the envelope protein of hepatitis B virus (the surface protein) and the polymerase protein. These two proteins use the same DNA sequence to encode different proteins but any change to the surface protein leads to a change in the polymerase protein. Hence hepatitis B virus cannot readily mutate its envelope (unlike hepatitis C virus) because many changes in the surface protein have an impact on the polymerase and lead to the production of non-functional viruses. Likewise only a few mutations in the polymerase protein are permitted since many changes lead to the generation of defective viral envelopes.

The replication of hepatitis B virus has been studied in tissue culture models, and the details are now well established (Fig. 4.2). The virus enters a cell and releases its partially double-stranded DNA genome. This genome is converted to covalently closed, circular DNA (cccDNA), which acts both as an infectious reservoir and as a template for replication. Some of the cccDNA remains in the nucleus, where it acts as a non-replicating viral repository that is unaffected by antiviral drugs. The remainder of the cccDNA is used to produce an RNA intermediate – the pregenomic RNA. This RNA is then reverse transcribed by the hepatitis B virus POL protein to produce new DNA that is ultimately duplicated and packaged into new viral particles.

During the replication cycle, new viral

Figure 4.1
A. Schematic diagram of the hepatitis B virus. The partially double-stranded DNA genome encodes four open reading frames. The surface gene contains three initiation codons that lead to the production of three different proteins (preS1, preS2 and surface protein) with different amino-terminals but a common carboxy-domain. These three proteins form both the envelope of the virus and the 'empty' virus particles (HBsAg). The core gene has two initiation codons that lead to the production of the core protein itself or a truncated, soluble version (HBeAg).

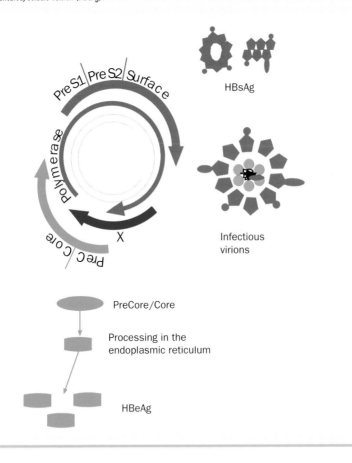

Figure 4.2

Replication of the hepatitis B virus. After entry into the cell (A) the virus is uncoated (B) and the partially double-stranded DNA is released (C). The partially double-stranded DNA is transported to the nucleus where it is converted to cccDNA. This cccDNA may remain in the nucleus to form a reservoir of non-replicating DNA, but most of the cccDNA is used as a template for the production of pre-genomic RNA. This pregenomic RNA acts as a template for the polymerase protein that converts the RNA into DNA (reverse transcription) before being destroyed by the polymerase-associated RNase. The new DNA is converted into the partially double stranded DNA form and then packaged into new virions before release (F and G)

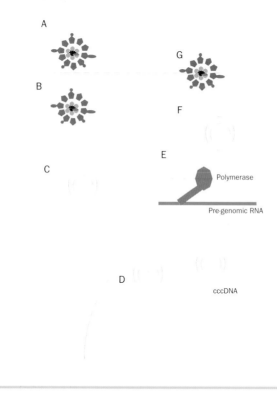

proteins are produced and combined to produce new virions. Some of the hepatitis B virus proteins are produced in excess and exported out of the cell to form circulating viral proteins that lack any viral nucleic acid. The hepatitis B virus surface protein is produced in vast excess and the released proteins form circulating particles whose function is not clear. These 'empty' viral particles, which contain only the hepatitis B virus surface proteins, are easily detected by standard laboratory assays and they form the basis of the hepatitis B virus surface antigen (HBsAg) diagnostic assay. Hence the assay that is widely used to detect hepatitis B virus infection actually identifies 'empty' viral shells and not the infectious virus.

The hepatitis B virus core protein is normally enclosed within the virus proper. However, the hepatitis B virus core gene can also be translated to produce a larger protein (precore–core), and this protein enters the endoplasmic reticulum, where it is cleaved to produce a smaller protein, HBeAg. This protein is secreted into the circulation, where it may be tolerogenic (see page 8). In clinical practice, HBeAg is a very useful marker of viral replication – its presence indicates that the virus is replicating at a high level and that the patient's serum will contain large numbers of infectious virions. In general, immune responses against HBeAg are associated with responses against other viral proteins and are associated with a reduction in the level of viral replication.

In addition to the two structural proteins (surface and core), the hepatitis B virus genome encodes two non-structural proteins – the X and POL proteins. The functions of the X protein are still unclear but it appears to play a role in regulating viral replication by controlling transcription of the viral genome. The complex POL protein contains the enzymes required for viral replication, including a reverse transcriptase and an RNase, and these combine to replicate the viral genome (see Fig. 4.2).

Natural history of chronic hepatitis B virus infection

The hepatitis B virus replicates almost exclusively in hepatocytes. Cells that are infected with the virus tolerate the infection remarkably well, and infected cells are usually not damaged by the virus. Hence many patients can sustain very large amounts of replicating virus without any significant liver injury.

Liver damage in patients with hepatitis B virus infection is therefore not due to the virus itself but to the immune response directed against hepatitis B virus – liver injury occurs only when there is an immune response against the virus.

Natural history of perinatally acquired chronic hepatitis B

The various phases of chronic hepatitis B virus infection are shown in Figure 4.3.

Immunotolerant phase of hepatitis B virus infection

In most countries, chronic hepatitis B virus infection is acquired early in life, either during birth or in the first few years of life. After infection, there is a reduced host response to the virus and the virus replicates at high level. It is not known why the host immune system does not recognize or respond to the presence of the virus but transplacental passage of HBeAg is believed to play a role in inducing a state of immunological tolerance in some patients. During this early 'immunotolerant' phase of hepatitis B virus infection, HBsAg and HBeAg are found in high concentration in the serum, and up to 10^9 copies/ml of hepatitis B virus DNA can be detected. Since there is no immune response against the virus there is no liver inflammation, and the liver function tests are usually normal or near normal.

> *The immunotolerant phase of hepatitis B virus infection can last for a few years or many decades.*

Immunoactive phase of hepatitis B virus infection

In most patients the immune system eventually recognizes the foreign virus and an immune response develops. This leads to an increase in liver cell damage (and an increase in serum aminotransferase levels). During this second phase – the immunoactive phase – the evolving immune response either controls the infection and the disease remits, or the immune response leads to a prolonged period of hepatic inflammation that often leads to a cirrhosis.

Hence, during the immunoactive phase the liver is either killed or cured! If the immune response against hepatitis B virus is sufficient to control the virus, there is often a brief increase in the hepatic inflammation during the elimination process, and this is usually associated with the loss of HBeAg and the development of antibodies against HBeAg. This 'seroconversion hepatitis' usually marks the transition from high-level viral replication to low-level viral replication, and the level of viraemia falls markedly (usually to less than 10^5 copies/ml serum). Although HBeAg is eliminated, HBsAg persists.

If the immune response fails to control the infection, there is a prolonged period of

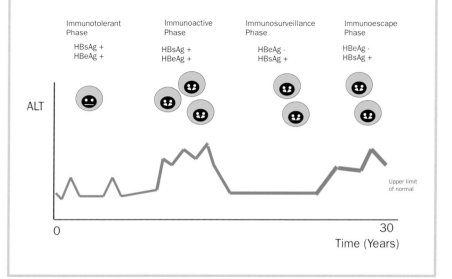

Figure 4.3
The natural history of chronic hepatitis B virus infection. Shortly after infection, the virus replicates at high levels, but there is no effective immune response (immunotolerance phase) and there is little hepatic damage. A variable time after infection, an immune response against the virus develops and leads to an increase in the severity of the liver damage, which may progress to cirrhosis at this stage. The immune response usually suppresses the viral replication, and the level of circulating viraemia declines and HBeAg is lost from the serum. This immunosurveillance phase may persist for many years but in some patients the virus mutates and disease develops once again.

fluctuating serum transaminase levels associated with increasing liver damage. The serum virological markers show that both HBsAg and HBeAg persist, and hepatitis B virus DNA may be detected at high levels (10^6–10^9 copies/ml). Since the liver injury is due to the immune response there is no correlation between the level of viraemia and the severity of the hepatitis.

Immunosurveillance phase of hepatitis B virus infection

If the immunoactive phase of hepatitis

B virus infection leads to control of the virus, the patient enters the immunosurveillance phase. During this phase of the infection the patient has:

- low levels of circulating virus;
- undetectable HBeAg; and
- readily detectable HBsAg.

Since the levels of circulating virus are low, the patient is of low infectivity and transmission of the virus to others is extremely rare. The patient may be regarded as having 'hepatitis B surface antigenaemia'. Patients in this phase of hepatitis B virus infection used to be referred to as 'chronic asymptomatic carriers'. However, since most phases of hepatitis B virus infection are asymptomatic and since patients during this phase of the infection are not actually carrying the virus the term is unhelpful and is best avoided.

The natural history of the immunosurveillance phase of chronic hepatitis B virus infection is not yet clear. A small proportion of patients go on to eliminate all traces of the virus and HBsAg eventually disappears from the serum along with all other circulating viral proteins. These patients may be regarded as 'cured', although severe

immunosuppression (e.g. during chemotherapy) may lead to a relapse.

Immunoescape chronic hepatitis B

Unfortunately, in a significant proportion of patients with hepatitis B surface antigenaemia, the virus becomes active again (immunoescape chronic hepatitis B). In these patients the level of hepatitis B virus DNA in the serum rises (usually above 10^5 copies/ml) and the hepatitis recurs with an increase in the level of the serum transaminases. The HBeAg remains undetectable and the antibodies against HBeAg persist. Careful analysis of the virus during this phase of the infection invariably reveals mutant viruses that lack the ability to produce HBeAg. The most common mutation causing this relapse is a mutation in the precore region that leads to a failure to produce the HBeAg. Hence this form of hepatitis B is often referred to as 'precore mutant hepatitis B'. However in some viral strains the precore mutant is unstable; in such strains mutations in the core promoter lead to the replication of viruses in the absence of HBeAg, so the term 'precore mutant hepatitis B' may be inaccurate and is probably best avoided.

HBeAg-negative active hepatitis B is becoming the dominant form of the disease in many Mediterranean countries, and its management is often problematic (see page 100).

Adult-acquired hepatitis B

Adults who are infected with the hepatitis B virus usually develop an acute, self-limiting illness. The patient becomes jaundiced and unwell, with upper abdominal pain. Joint aches are common. In most patients the illness resolves without sequelae, but in a small minority (2%) the disease leads on to acute liver failure (fulminant hepatitis). Early detection of acute liver failure is essential for successful management (usually by transplantation), and the progress of acute hepatitis B virus infection should be monitored by regular assessment of the prothrombin index and the serum albumin concentration (since serum aminotransferase levels may be misleading in this setting).

Acute hepatitis B virus infection requires no treatment, but contacts should be protected by appropriate vaccination.

Occasionally adults who contract hepatitis B develop chronic infection, which progresses as outlined above.

Pathology of hepatitis B virus infection

Acute hepatitis

Patients with acute hepatitis B rarely undergo liver biopsy. If a biopsy is performed it is either in error or because the associated liver disease is so severe that the patient is being considered for transplantation. The histological picture is, as with all aetiologies of acute hepatitis, characterized by 'spotty' necrosis. Immunohistochemical staining may demonstrate HBsAg or hepatitis B virus core antigen (HBcAg), but ground glass cells are not seen – their presence is pathognomonic of chronic hepatitis B.

Chronic hepatitis

General features of chronic hepatitis B virus infection

The essential histological features of chronic hepatitis B (Table 4.1) infection are the same as for all aetiologies of chronic hepatitis:

- chronic inflammation that involves the portal tracts, the limiting plate (interface hepatitis or 'piecemeal necrosis') and lobules; and
- fibrosis of the portal tracts, which may range from portal tract expansion to cirrhosis.

Table 4.1
Specific histological features in chronic hepatitis B virus infection

Immunocompetent patients
Ground glass hepatocytes
Immunopathic hepatocyte damage

Immunosuppressed patients
Fibrosing cholestatic hepatitis

Although lymphoid follicles may be seen
in hepatitis B, they are much less
common and tend to be much less well
developed than in hepatitis C. As in
chronic hepatitis C, the inflammatory
changes determine the grade of disease
and the fibrotic changes determine the
stage of disease. The severity of the
disease can be assessed using one of a
number of semiquantitative scoring
systems (see page 35).

On conventionally stained sections, two
features are characteristic of chronic
hepatitis B virus infection:

- ground glass hepatocytes; and
- evidence of immunopathic liver cell
  damage.

Ground glass cells (Figs 4.4, 4.5 and 4.6)
contain finely granular cytoplasm, often
with an artefactual halo around them. It is
salutary for histopathologists to remember
that these cells were first described by a

physician! They contain large amounts of
HBsAg secondary to integration of
hepatitis B virus DNA into the genome of
the cell and its subsequent transcription.
Ground glass cells can be demonstrated by
histochemical techniques (Gamori's
aldehyde fuschin, orcein or Victoria blue
stain) or by immunohistochemical
techniques.

There are other, unusual causes of ground
glass cells, the most common of which is
induction of the smooth endoplasmic
reticulum by enzyme-inducing drugs;
other causes include Lafora bodies in
myoclonic epilepsy and fibrinogen storage
disease.

Ground glass also need to be distinguished
from cells showing oxyntic change.
Oxyntic change can be seen both in
chronic hepatitis B and hepatitis C (Fig.
4.7). It is a form of cellular degeneration
in which the cells come to contain large
numbers of closely packed mitochondria.

In the very rare cases in which ground
glass hepatocytes on liver biopsy are seen
but in which the patient is serum HBsAg-
negative, immunohistochemical staining is
useful. Ground glass cells are especially
prominent in patients with
immunotolerant hepatitis B with relatively
inactive disease. In the immunoactive

Figure 4.4
Liver with scattered
ground glass hepatocytes
(arrowed). These cells
have finely granular
cytoplasm with
artefactual halos.

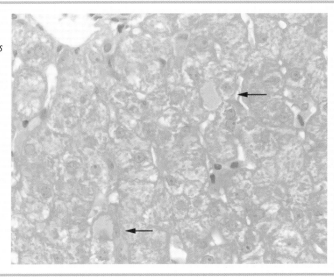

Figure 4.5
Liver stained with an
orcein stain, which
highlights ground glass
hepatocytes caused by
hepatitis B virus infection.

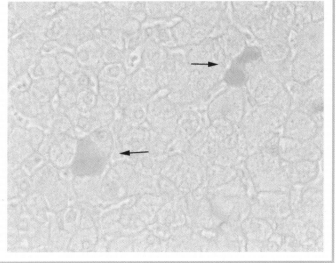

Figure 4.6
Immunohistochemical stain for HbsAg, which confirms that the ground glass change is due to the accumulation of HBsAg in the cytoplasm.

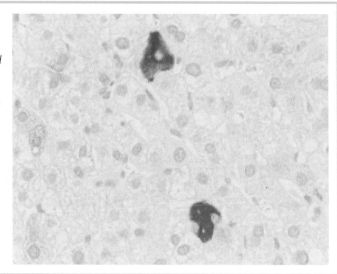

Figure 4.7
Hepatocytes with intensely pink granular cytoplasm caused by the accumulation of large numbers of mitochondria. This change can be seen in many types of liver damage.

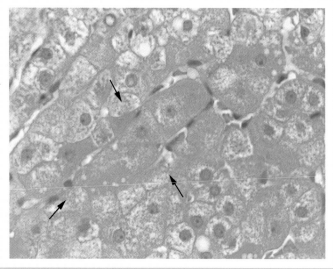

phase of chronic hepatitis B, the liver damage is due to immunological injury by cytotoxic CD8-positive T lymphocytes that recognize HBeAg or HBcAg on the surface of infected hepatocytes in association with HLA class 1 antigens (see page 6). The histological correlate of this is that lymphocytes are often seen in close relation to damaged hepatocytes.

The presence of marked lobular inflammation and cytopathic liver cell damage with hepatocytes that show acidophilic degeneration in a patient with chronic hepatitis B should always raise the possibility of a superimposed hepatitis delta virus infection (see page 103).

Chronic hepatitis B virus infection is frequently associated with dysplasia, which is a marker for an increased risk of developing liver cell cancer (see page 150). Given the frequency of hepatitis B virus infection in certain ethnic groups, the presence of another cause of liver disease should always be considered. The exclusion of other causes of liver disease is one reason why all patients with chronic viral hepatitis should have at least one liver biopsy.

Immunohistochemical features of chronic hepatitis B virus infection

A wide range of commercially available antibodies to hepatitis B virus are available. While there are cases in which immunohistochemical staining of liver biopsies is valuable, such cases are uncommon and many laboratories frequently carry out staining for hepatitis B virus antigens unnecessarily. This is because immunohistochemical staining rarely provides information not already available from serology. There are a number of circumstances in which immunohistochemical staining can be useful; these are discussed below and summarized in Table 4.2. As discussed above, cytoplasmic HBsAg staining is seen in ground glass hepatocytes. Membranous and submembranous staining can also be seen (see Fig. 4.5). Membranous staining correlates with active viral replication. Both HBcAg and HBeAg produce nuclear staining with and without cytoplasmic staining (Figs 4.8 and 4.9). The latter also correlates with active viral replication. It should be noted that the pattern of HBcAg and HBeAg staining can be used as a means of assessing disease activity, although this is not part of routine clinical practice. There is also no clinical role for *in situ* hybridization to demonstrate hepatitis B virus DNA. It should be noted

Table 4.2
Indications for immunohistochemical staining in hepatitis B virus infection

To investigate possible cases of HBeAg negative chronic hepatitis B
To exclude co-existing hepatitis delta virus infection
To exclude hepatitis B virus infection as a cause of lobular hepatitis in an immunosuppressed patient
To confirm the aetiology of ground glass hepatocytes (rare)

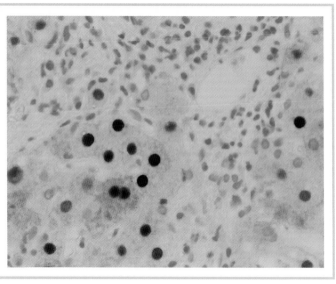

Figure 4.8
Liver biopsy from a patient with hepatitis B stained immunohistochemically with an antibody to HBeAg. The predominantly intranuclear staining is characteristic of relatively inactive disease. The presence of HBeAg also confirms the presence of wild type virus.

that hepatitis B virus DNA can sometimes be identified in the liver in patients who are negative for hepatitis B virus DNA in the serum.

Pathology of the immunotolerant phase of hepatitis B virus infection

The immunotolerant phase is the early phase of chronic hepatitis B virus infection, when the immune response is inadequate and liver damage is mild.

Figure 4.9
Liver biopsy from a patient with HBV stained immunohistochemically with an antibody to HBeAg. The widespread intranuclear and cytoplasmic staining indicates active viral replication.

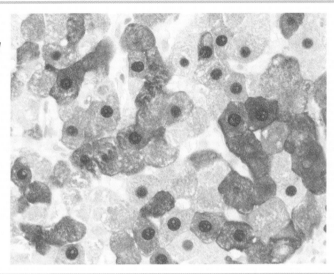

Patients in this phase respond poorly to treatment, and the clinician should be advised to withhold therapy and monitor the patient (see page 94).

The histological features of the immunotolerant phase include:

- large numbers of ground glass hepatocytes; and
- mild fibrous expansion of portal tracts with mild portal and lobular inflammation.

Even at this early stage, large cell dysplasia may be seen (see page 150).

Pathology of the immunoactive phase of hepatitis B virus infection

In the immunoactive phase of chronic hepatitis B virus infection, an immune response against the virus leads to significant liver damage. Patients in this phase of the disease are likely to develop progressive liver disease and are likely to benefit from therapy – hence therapy is appropriate at this time.

The histological features include:

- architectural changes ranging from fibrous expansion of portal tracts and necroinflammatory changes (e.g. mild

or moderate portal inflammation, interface hepatitis, lobular inflammation); and
• possibly dysplasia.

Ground glass cells are relatively uncommon. Since immunoactive hepatitis B virus infection with cirrhosis may respond poorly to therapy, it is important to alert the clinician if features of cirrhosis are present.

Pathology of the immunosurveillance phase of chronic hepatitis B virus infection

In the immunosurveillance phase of infection, the virus replicates at very low levels and HBsAg and the antibody against HBeAg are found in the serum. Typically the liver function tests are normal, and a liver biopsy is rarely performed. However, deciding whether a patient has HBeAg-negative chronic hepatitis B (see page 129) or merely hepatitis B surface antigenaemia can be extremely difficult. The viral serology is the same in these two conditions, but in HBeAg-negative chronic hepatitis B liver damage is likely and in hepatitis B surface antigenaemia no injury is expected.

In most patients the diagnosis is straightforward – the liver function tests are normal in patients with isolated hepatitis B surface antigenaemia and abnormal in patients with HBeAg-negative chronic hepatitis B. However, in some patients with HBeAg-negative chronic hepatitis B, the liver function tests fluctuate although they may be normal for many months. To make diagnosis even more difficult, the level of hepatitis B virus DNA in the serum in the two disorders may overlap – typically patients with HBeAg-negative disease have a high level of hepatitis B virus DNA (more than 10^5/ml) and patients with hepatitis B surface antigenaemia have a lower level. However, in HBeAg-negative disease the levels of hepatitis B virus DNA may fluctuate, and some patients with isolated hepatitis B surface antigenaemia have relatively high levels of hepatitis B virus DNA.

Hence, distinguishing between the two can be very difficult, and the liver biopsy may be very helpful in this setting (Table 4.3). The typical histological features in hepatitis B surface antigenaemia include:

• variable degrees of fibrosis;
• mild necroinflammation;
• ground glass hepatocytes; and
• dysplasia (possibly).

Table 4.3
A typical liver biopsy report from a patient with hepatitis B virus infection

---

Macroscopic appearance
Fragments of brown tissue 2.5 cm in aggregate length
Microscopic appearance
Liver with cirrhotic architecture
There is moderate portal inflammation and interface hepatitis
The bile ducts are normal
There is mild lobular inflammation and ground glass hepatocytes are present
Special stains for iron, alpha-1 antitrypsin bodies and copper-associated protein are negative
There is focal large cell dysplasia
Conclusion
An active cirrhosis with dysplasia due to hepatitis B virus infection
Modified HAI score
Grade – 2+0+1+2=5/18
Stage – 6/6

Pathology of immunoescape chronic hepatitis B (HBeAg-negative chronic hepatitis B)

In this late phase of infection, mutant hepatitis B virus causes liver damage despite the presence of an immune response directed against the virus. The typical histological features include all the features seen in the immunoactive phase.

In all patients who are HBeAg negative but who have active histological disease the possibility of the patient having developed the mutant virus must be considered. On immunohistochemical staining patients with HBeAg-negative chronic infection show positive staining for HBcAg but are negative for HBeAg. The presence of hepatic HBeAg correlates with circulating wild type virus.

Histological features in immunosuppressed patients

Hepatitis B is occasionally seen in patients with HIV infection and may occur in patients who are immunosuppressed (e.g. as recurrent disease in patients who have had a liver transplant for chronic hepatitis B). Since hepatitis B is an immunopathic virus, in immunosuppressed patients necroinflammatory activity is usually low, although there is associated active viral replication. On the other hand, in HIV-positive patients improvement in the

CD4-positive T-cell counts following highly active anti-retroviral therapy may be associated with a marked increase in liver damage. In some patients who have cleared the hepatitis B virus and who are HBeAg-negative, or even HBsAg-negative, immunosuppression may be associated with reactivation of viral infection. The histological picture in these patients is that of a lobular (acute) hepatitis. This group of patients includes patients with haematological malignancies being treated with cytotoxic agents. The presence of a lobular hepatitis in an immunosuppressed patient is, therefore, an indication for immunohistochemical staining for hepatitis B virus as well as for cytomegalovirus and other viruses.

A particular form of liver damage was first described in patients who had recurrent hepatitis B virus in their grafted livers – fibrosing cholestatic hepatitis. It is characterized by rapidly progressive liver cell fibrosis associated with bile duct proliferation and liver cell damage. A very similar condition has been reported in a small number of patients with hepatitis B virus infection who have received a renal transplant or who have AIDS. This condition appears to be caused by the exceptionally high viral loads that can be seen in the livers

of these patients and the resulting cytopathic liver cell damage.

In immunosuppressed patients, immunohistochemical staining for HBsAg and HBeAg and should always be carried out if there is no other obvious cause for the liver damage seen. This is true both in patients with a lobular hepatitis and in those with a fibrosis and bile duct proliferation.

Further reading

Carmen W, Jacyna M, Hadziyannis S, *et al*. Mutation preventing formation of e antigen in patients with chronic HBV infection. *Lancet* 1989; **2**: 588–91.

Chisari FV, Ferrari C. Hepatitis B virus immunopathogenesis. *Annu Rev Immunol* 1995; **13**: 29–60.

Ganem D. The molecular biology of the hepatitis B virus. *Annu Rev Biochem* 1987; **56**: 651–93

Liaw Y, Chu C, Su I, Huang M, Lin D, Chang C. Clinical and histological events preceeding hepatitis B e antigen seroconversion in chronic Type B hepatitis. *Gastroenterology* 1983; **84**: 216–19.

Lok A, Lai C. Acute exacerbations in Chinese patients with chronic hepatitis B virus infection: incidence, predisposing factors and etiology. *J Hepatol* 1990; **10**: 29–34.

Lok AS, Liang RHS, Chiu EKW, *et al.* Reactivation of hepatitis B virus replication in patients receiving cytotoxic therapy. *Gastroenterology* 1991; **100**: 182–8.

Mills CT, Lee E, Perrillo R: Relationship between histologic, aminotransferase levels, and viral replication in chronic hepatitis B. *Gastroenterology* 1990; **99**: 519–24.

Perrillo RP, Brunt EM. Hepatic histologic and immunohistochemical changes in chronic hepatitis B after prolonged clearance of hepatitis B e antigen and hepatitis B surface antigen. *Ann Intern Med* 1991; **115**: 113–15.

Questions

1. Regarding the hepatitis B virus:
   A. The X protein crosses the placenta and induces a state of tolerance
   B. The reverse transcriptase enzyme is similar to the HIV enzyme, and some drugs act in both diseases
   C. Elimination of the cccDNA is required to clear all replicating forms

D. The surface protein is produced in vast excess
E. HBeAg is encoded by the same gene that codes for the core protein

2. During chronic hepatitis B virus infection:
   A. The immunotolerant phase is characterized by high levels of virus and severe liver damage
   B. The seroconversion reaction involves loss of HBeAg and the development of antibodies against HBeAg, and it is clinically silent
   C. If HBeAg is not detected in serum, any liver disease that is present cannot be due to hepatitis B virus
   D. The severity of the liver damage is not necessarily dependent on the levels of viral replication
   E. Adult infection usually leads to an acute infection

3. In a liver biopsy from a patient with chronic hepatitis B:
   A. The ground glass hepatocytes are a unique feature of chronic hepatitis B virus infection
   B. Immunohostochemical staining is of no value
   C. Interface hepatitis (piecemeal necrosis) indicates autoimmune liver disease
   D. Lymphocytes are typically associated

with hepatocytes since the liver disease is due to immune-mediated destruction of infected cells

E. Dysplastic hepatocytes may indicate that the patient has an increased risk of developing liver cell cancer

4. The following may help to distinguish between the immunosurveillance phase of hepatitis B (hepatitis B surface antigenaemia) and HBeAg-negative chronic hepatitis B:
    A. Serum HBV DNA levels
    B. Titre of IgM anticore antibodies
    C. Immunohistochemistry of a liver biopsy specimen
    D. The titre of HBsAg
    E. The liver function tests

Answers

Question 1

A. False – the HBeAg behaves in this way
B. True
C. True
D. True
E. True

Question 2

A. False – during the immunotolerant phase the virus replicates at high levels

but the absence of an immune response ensures that the liver damage is mild

B. False – this seroconversion reaction is usually associated with an increase in the severity of the hepatitis

C. False – HBeAg-negative chronic hepatitis B is associated with significant liver injury

D. True
E. True

Question 3

A. False – a number of other conditions can also give rise to ground glass cells

B. False – immunohistochemistry may aid in distinguishing between the immunosurveillance phase of chronic hepatitis B and the HBeAg-negative chronic hepatitis B

C. False – it may be seen in a number of chronic liver diseases including viral hepatitis and primary biliary cirrhosis

D. True
E. True

Question 4

A. True
B. True
C. True
D. False
E. True

Management of chronic hepatitis B virus infection

5

Chronic hepatitis B virus infection is extremely common, and patients present at all stages of the disease.

The diagnosis and management is based on an understanding of its natural history, which is discussed in Chapter 4.

Diagnosis

Patients with chronic hepatitis B virus infection are typically referred when a virology laboratory reports the presence of HBsAg in serum. For such patients, a full hepatitis B virological profile should be performed with assessment of:

- the HBeAg status and antibodies against HBeAg;
- the HBcAg status; and
- liver function tests.

The results of these investigations should be reviewed to determine both the nature and the phase of the infection.

The first step is to determine whether the infection is acute or chronic. A history of recent exposure to the virus (via sexual or other contact) with jaundice, malaise and markedly abnormal liver function tests (transaminase levels over 500 IU/ml) is suggestive of an acute infection, and this is usually confirmed by the finding of a high titre of IgM antibodies to the HBcAg (IgM HBcAb). Although the presence of IgM HBcAb is usually regarded as proof of an acute infection, these antibodies may also develop during activation of a chronic infection (i.e. during conversion from the immunotolerant to the immunoactive phase), and therefore the presence of IgM antibodies should be regarded as strongly suggestive of an acute infection and not as proof of recent infection. During an acute hepatitis B virus infection, the virological markers of infection change rapidly and thus all or no antigens may be present (HBsAg and HBeAg) and antibodies against hepatitis B virus may or may not be identified.

Once acute infection has been excluded, the phase of the hepatitis B virus infection should be determined by examining the HBeAg status. If HBeAg is detected in serum then the patient is viraemic and the liver function tests should be examined.

If the liver function tests are normal or near normal, the patient is most likely to be in the immunotolerant phase of the disease, and therapy should be withheld until there is evidence of activity. Measurement of the level of viraemia in these patients is usually of little diagnostic value – if measured, the serum hepatitis B virus DNA concentration is likely to be high (often around 10^7–10^9 copies/ml). A liver biopsy at this stage is helpful to exclude cirrhosis and to confirm the phase of the disease.

If the liver function tests are markedly abnormal then immunoactive disease is likely. A liver biopsy should be performed to confirm the diagnosis and to exclude cirrhosis. Early therapy should be considered. Once again, assessment of the viral load is unlikely to be of diagnostic or therapeutic value, and high hepatitis B virus DNA levels are to be expected.

Patients who are HBeAg-negative should be assessed to determine whether there is residual virus and disease activity (HBeAg-negative disease) or whether the patient simply has persisting hepatitis B virus surface antigenaemia. As discussed in Chapter 4, it can be surprisingly difficult to distinguish between these two forms of disease. The liver function tests provide most diagnostic information in this setting – if they are normal, persisting hepatitis B virus surface antigenaemia is probable and the patient is unlikely to develop further disease. If the hepatitis B virus DNA level is measured directly it is found to be low or undetectable (usually less than 10^4 copies/ml); however, this measurement is not usually required in these patients.

Patients with persisting hepatitis B virus surface antigenamia are often discharged from further follow-up. In our view it is prudent to keep these patients under distant review, and we monitor all such patients every year to identify late disease reactivation.

The identification of patients with HBeAg-negative chronic hepatitis B is usually made by examining the liver function tests. If the liver function tests are abnormal the most likely diagnosis is the presence of mutant hepatitis B virus that does not produce HBeAg (HBeAg-negative disease). This diagnosis should be confirmed by measuring the hepatitis B virus DNA levels, which will be elevated (more than 10^5 copies/ml), and alternative diagnoses (e.g. hepatitis delta virus superinfection, drug reactions) should be considered and excluded by a careful history and a liver biopsy.

Some patients with HBeAg-negative chronic hepatitis B have relapsing–remitting disease in which the liver function tests are normal for long periods of time but occasionally relapse with an acute hepatitis-like picture. During the quiescent period the hepatitis B virus DNA levels may be very low but they are usually elevated just before a disease flare. This unusual form of chronic hepatitis B can usually be identified by careful observation over a period of several months but, because the hepatitic flares (when the liver function tests are elevated and the hepatitis B virus DNA levels are raised) may be transient, identification can be difficult. In the hepatitic flares that are common in HBeAg-negative chronic hepatitis B, the IgM HBcAb titre is often raised, and this increase may persist for some months. This has led some to suggest that detecting high levels of IgM HBcAb should be used routinely to diagnose HBeAg-negative chronic hepatitis B, but the sensitivity and specificity of this approach have not been rigorously tested.

The HBeAg-negative form of hepatitis B was first identified by genome sequencing of the hepatitis B virus precore region in patients with active liver disease and undetectable HBeAg. A single nucleotide substitution at position 1896 was found in these patients and has since been reported in a high proportion of patients with HBeAg-negative disease. It is tempting to use the identification of this mutation as a diagnostic tool for the HBeAg-negative form of hepatitis B, and many groups have used viral sequencing in an effort to predict who will go on to develop HBeAg-negative disease. These studies have shown that a high proportion of patients with 'normal' virus (i.e. HBeAg-positive chronic hepatitis B) carry the mutant virus and many of them eventually eliminate all traces of the virus. Hence the presence of the mutant virus cannot be used to predict who will develop HBeAg-negative disease. In patients who have HBeAg-negative chronic hepatitis B, sequencing of the precore region may reveal the presence of the 1896 mutation. However, many patients develop other mutations that lead to the same phenotype and thus routine sequencing of the genome of hepatitis B is of no diagnostic or therapeutic value.

An algorithm for the diagnosis of hepatitis B is shown in Figure 5.1.

One of the most difficult problems in the diagnosis of chronic hepatitis B is distinguishing between hepatitis B surface antigenaemia and HBeAg-negative chronic hepatitis B. Many patients who are HBsAg-

positive and HBeAg-negative are referred for advice and therapy, and the majority have simple hepatitis B surface antigenaemia that requires no further action. A minority have HBeAg-negative disease but this rare condition may only be diagnosed by regular review over many months, with at least one liver biopsy. The clinician is faced with the problem of how to investigate the patient appropriately while avoiding unnecessary investigations.

Since HBeAg-negative disease is rare in Africa and Asia, it is reasonable not to perform intensive monitoring in patients of African or Asian descent who have normal liver function tests in the presence of HBsAg and HBeAb in the serum. We review these patients every year.

In Mediterranean countries, HBeAg-negative disease is now quite common and we believe that more intensive monitoring is appropriate. We review such patients every 3 months for the first year and, if the liver function tests become abnormal during this time, we perform hepatitis B virus DNA assays and a liver biopsy. If the liver function tests remain normal during this year of intensive monitoring, we review the patient on an annual basis.

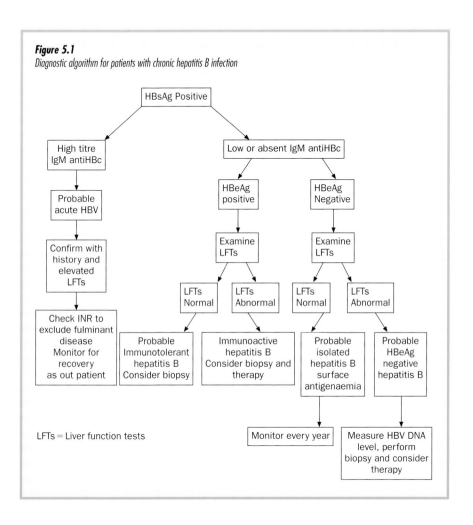

Figure 5.1
Diagnostic algorithm for patients with chronic hepatitis B infection

LFTs = Liver function tests

Management of the patient with chronic hepatitis B virus infection

Prevention of transmission

All patients who have evidence of ongoing hepatitis B virus infection are at risk of transmitting the virus to others. The risk is greatest in those who are HBeAg-positive or who have high-level viraemia (more than 10^5 copies/ml), but even those who are HBeAg-negative with low level viraemia may, albeit rarely, transmit the infection.

> *Since vaccination to prevent hepatitis B virus infection is safe and well tolerated, all contacts of infected patients should be protected by vaccination and, in many countries routine hepatitis B vaccination of such contacts is provided.*

> *The hepatitis B virus is highly infectious and is readily transmitted by blood products, sexual contact or passage from mother to baby during childbirth – all who are infected should be warned about the risks of transmission and advised to practice safe sex and to arrange for regular partners to be vaccinated.*

The standard hepatitis B vaccine uses HBsAg particles produced in yeast, and the vaccine is well tolerated and safe. The vast majority of vaccinated people respond well, but a small proportion (5%) do not respond; in those at high risk of infection (e.g. close contacts of infected patients) it is therefore prudent to check the effectiveness of the vaccination schedule by assessing the antibody response (by measuring the titre of antibodies against HBsAg) 6 months after the last injection. A titre of more than 10 iu/ml is protective but most authorities recommend that the antibody titre should be maintained at more than 100 iu/ml (see Chapter 1 for further discussion of the value of monitoring the antibody response).

For high-risk people who have shown a partial response to the vaccine (i.e. those who have developed low antibody titres), further injections of the standard vaccine are recommended, but for those who have shown no response at all, further innoculations are unlikely to be of benefit. For such vaccine 'non-responders' there is currently no effective vaccine although new modified vaccines are being developed and may be available in the future.

Active vaccination against hepatitis B virus is effective but the antibodies are produced only a few months after inoculation. For unprotected people who have been exposed to hepatitis B virus, passive vaccination with anti-hepatitis B serum (HBIg) should be considered

(Table 5.1). This expensive prophylaxis should be reserved for those who have had significant contact with the virus and are not already protected by vaccination (e.g. medical personnel exposed to a needle stick injury who have not responded to the standard vaccine). HBIg is widely used for children born to HBeAg-positive mothers; it is given to the newborn baby immediately after birth in association with active vaccination, usually in the contralateral arm.

Although the current vaccines against hepatitis B virus protect most people from infection, a tiny proportion of vaccinated people become infected with hepatitis B virus despite the presence of antibodies against the standard vaccine. Analysis of the virus in these people shows that they are usually infected with a mutant virus (a 'vaccine-escape' mutant) that changes the structure of the envelope protein such that antibodies against the vaccine do not neutralize the viruses. These mutant strains of hepatitis B are rare but there is concern that the increasing use of current vaccines will lead to the widespread development of vaccine-resistant strains.

Therapy for patients with chronic hepatitis B virus infection

All patients with chronic hepatitis B virus infection should receive appropriate counselling about:

- infectivity; viral transmission; and
- possible therapeutic interventions.

> *Appropriate selection of patients is a prerequisite for successful therapy, and an accurate assessment of the stage of disease by liver biopsy is essential before therapy.*

Table 5.1
Vaccination schedules for hepatitis B

The vaccine should be administered by intramuscular injection into the deltoid muscle (the vaccine is less effective when administered into the buttock):

Standard vaccination:
0   Month 1   Month 6

Accelerated vaccination:
0   Month 1   Month 2   Month 12

Therapeutic options
There are two broad approaches to therapy in patients with chronic hepatitis B virus infection:

- immunostimulation with a 3-month course of interferon; and
- prolonged suppression of viral replication with a reverse transcriptase inhibitor such as lamivudine.

Long-term suppression with lamivudine often leads to the development of an immune response against hepatitis B virus and the disease moves into the immunosurveillance phase (hepatitis B surface antigenaemia), with permanent loss of HBeAg and the development of antibodies against this protein. Since lamivudine therapy is well tolerated, most patients prefer this approach to therapy.

Timing of therapy in patients with HBeAg-positive chronic hepatitis B

During the early phase of chronic hepatitis B virus infection (the immunotolerant phase with high-level viraemia and normal liver function tests), there is no effective immune response against the virus, and immunostimulation with interferon is almost always ineffective and should be avoided. Therapy with lamivudine leads to suppression of viraemia but, since there is no pre-existing immune response, the virus is not eliminated and there is a high risk of the development of lamivudine-resistant mutants (see page 98). Hence, during the immunotolerant phase of chronic hepatitis B virus infection, therapy is not recommended – patients should be advised that their liver is not being damaged, and liver function tests should be monitored every 6 months. Any increase in the transaminase level should

prompt an increase in the intensity of monitoring and, if the increase in liver inflammation (i.e. increased alanine aminotransferase) is maintained for more than 3 months, it is likely that the disease has moved into the second phase, the immunoactive phase. Patients with immunoactive hepatitis B should undergo therapy.

During the immunoactive phase of chronic hepatitis B virus infection there is an ongoing immune response, and therapy may lead to seroconversion (i.e. the development of antibodies against HBeAg) and a marked reduction in circulating viraemia. Treatment with lamivudine (100 mg/day) for 1 year leads to seroconversion in up to 30% of these patients and, if therapy is prolonged for a further 3 years, up to 75% can be expected to seroconvert. Therapy with interferon-alpha (at a dose of 9 Miu three times a week) leads to seroconversion in 30–40% of patients, but the therapy is unpleasant (interferon has to be given by subcutaneous injection and induces malaise, depression and bone marrow suppression), and most patients prefer to receive oral therapy with daily lamivudine. However, although lamivudine is very well tolerated, it has to be taken every day for a prolonged period and some patients prefer to suffer the side effects of interferon

Table 5.2
Comparison between interferon and lamivudine therapy for immunoactive chronic hepatitis B

	Lamivudine	Interferon
Duration of therapy	1–4 years	3 months
Mode of administration	Oral tablet	Subcutaneous injection
Efficacy	20–30% after 1 year of treatment; >70% after 4 years of treatment	30–40% after 3 months of treatment
Side effects	Virtually none	Flu-like illness Nausea Hair loss Bone marrow suppression

therapy for 3 months rather than to undergo regular medication. These issues should be discussed with the patient. Lamivudine and interferon therapy for immunoactive chronic hepatitis B are compared in Table 5.2.

Management of patients receiving lamivudine therapy for chronic hepatitis B virus infection
Patients who elect to undergo therapy with lamivudine should have a liver biopsy performed before starting therapy. The biopsy should be assessed to exclude other causes for the abnormal liver function tests and should exclude cirrhosis. Lamivudine therapy is not contraindicated in patients with hepatitis B-related cirrhosis, but therapy in

advanced disease requires careful consideration since the development of lamivudine resistance may hinder transplantation (see page 130).

In patients with biopsy-proven immunoactive hepatitis B and no evidence of cirrhosis, lamivudine therapy should be started at a dose of 100 mg/day. Patients should be advised not to discontinue their medication for any reason and should be assessed every 3 months. At subsequent visits, the hepatitis B virology should be assessed along with the liver function tests. Within a few days of commencing lamivudine therapy the hepatitis B virus DNA level falls dramatically and the liver function tests normalize. With continued therapy there is an increasing chance of the development of a seroconversion reaction in which HBeAg disappears and HBeAb develop. Once a seroconversion reaction has developed and matured (i.e. once HBeAg is undetectable and HBeAb are present) therapy may safely be discontinued. At this stage the patient has moved to the immunosurveillance phase of infection and should be reviewed every year to ensure that HBeAg-negative chronic hepatitis B does not develop.

During therapy with lamivudine there is a small risk of the development of lamivudine-resistant mutations. These are point mutations in the polymerase gene of the hepatitis B virus that are associated with a reduction in the sensitivity of the virus to lamivudine. The mutations often, but not always, lead to the development of a YMDD protein motif in the polymerase protein; this mutant does not bind to the drug but is capable of sustaining viral replication. The development of these mutations can often be identified clinically by the development of abnormal liver function tests and by an associated increase in hepatitis B virus DNA. The diagnosis can be confirmed by direct sequencing of the virus, although this is rarely required. If a patient receiving lamivudine does develop a lamivudine-resistant mutation, the therapy must be

continued. It is now clear that the 'lamivudine resistant virus' replicates less well than the parental strain and the mutant virus seems to be associated with less liver damage. If lamivudine is continued there is a high probability of a seroconversion reaction and viral clearance even though the mutant hepatitis B virus is present at low levels.

Management of patients receiving interferon therapy for chronic hepatitis B virus infection

Patients who decide to undergo interferon therapy for chronic hepatitis B virus infection should also have a liver biopsy performed. Again this helps to confirm the diagnosis and excludes the presence of cirrhosis, which increases the risk of severe complications developing (see page 129). As with patients receiving interferon therapy for chronic hepatitis C (see page 55), a careful pretreatment assessment is essential. The patient should be assessed for previous psychiatric problems that may increase the likelihood of severe depression while receiving interferon, and a full blood count should be performed. Interferon therapy is likely to reduce the platelet and white cell counts and, in general, the platelet count should be greater than 70 and the neutrophil count should exceed 1×10^9 cells/l before starting therapy.

Treatment with interferon should be

started at a dose of 9 Miu three times a week (i.e. at a much higher dose than that used in patients with chronic hepatitis C) and continued for a total of 3 months. The full blood count and liver function tests should be monitored carefully throughout therapy (weekly for the first month and monthly thereafter), and the dose of interferon should be reduced if there is significant bone marrow suppression. Routine measurement of hepatitis B virus DNA is not required but it is helpful to measure the liver function tests during therapy. The serum transaminases usually normalize during the first few days of therapy and may then increase markedly during the third month. This increase in hepatic inflammation (hepatic flare) usually indicates that an immune response against the virus has developed and is often associated with the loss of HBeAg and the development of antibodies against hepatitis B virus. It usually indicates that therapy will be successful, although in patients with advanced cirrhosis the seroconversion hepatitis may lead to hepatic decompensation and therefore the liver function (serum albumin and prothrombin index) should be carefully assessed during therapy in these patients.

In some patients, a seroconversion reaction develops during interferon therapy (typically during the third month) and the disease moves from the immunoactive to the immunosurveillance phase. For these patients, annual review is recommended to detect any late relapse. However, in many patients there is no immune response against the virus during therapy, the liver function tests do not rise markedly and, when interferon therapy is stopped, the serum transaminases often become abnormal once again. For these patients ('non-responders') there is the possibility of a late response, since a seroconversion reaction may develop in the months after interferon therapy. We usually follow patients for 6 months after failed interferon therapy before considering alternative approaches (usually lamivudine therapy).

In many viral infections (e.g. hepatitis C virus and HIV), combination therapy significantly improves the response to therapy, and attempts have been made to improve the therapy of chronic hepatitis B by combining interferon and lamivudine. Trials to date, rather surprisingly, have shown no synergistic effect, but it is possible that further studies will identify circumstances in which the two drugs do synergize. For the present, combination therapy with lamivudine and interferon cannot be recommended.

Treatment of HBeAg-negative chronic hepatitis B

Management of patients with HBeAg-negative chronic hepatitis B is unsatisfactory. Since an effective immune response has already occurred (as shown by the presence of antibodies against HBeAg), further immunostimulation is unlikely to be helpful and, indeed, a 3-month course of high-dose interferon therapy in these patients is of little value. Prolonged therapy of at least 12 months with low-dose interferon-alpha (3–5 Miu three times a week) has been shown to induce a sustained response (i.e. no recurrence of disease or viraemia after 12 months) in up to 20% of treated patients. Thus HBeAg-negative chronic hepatitis B virus infection seems to behave like chronic hepatitis C virus infection in that prolonged low-dose interferon therapy is required to induce a cure in the minority. Trials with the new pegylated interferons in HBeAg-negative chronic hepatitis B are currently under consideration.

Treatment of HBeAg-negative chronic hepatitis B with lamivudine appears to be beneficial in the short term – the viraemia declines and the liver function tests improve. However, if the therapy is discontinued after 1 year the virus almost invariably recurs. Prolonged therapy leads to the development of lamivudine resistance and return of viraemia, and

after 3 years of therapy up to 50% of treated patients have developed lamivudine-resistant mutants. In these patients in whom an immunological viral clearance is not possible, the development of lamivudine resistance is not associated with eventual viral clearance, and the emergence of resistant viral strains may be associated with further progression of the liver damage. Some studies have reported the development of marked hepatitis associated with the development of lamivudine-resistant mutants but the frequency with which this occurs is not known.

Novel reverse transcripatase inhibitors are currently being evaluated. The most promising compound at present is adefovir depixol. This oral agent is a potent inhibitor of hepatitis B virus replication and acts against the lamivudine-resistant variants both *in vitro* and *in vivo*. It is likely that combination therapy with lamivudine and adefovir will prove to be effective in patients with HBeAg-negative chronic hepatitis B but further clinical trials will be needed to confirm that this is the case.

At present, there is no effective therapy for HBeAg-negative chronic hepatitis B, and further progress is unlikely until more reverse transcriptase inhibitors are available. For patients who are stable with mild fibrosis, therapy is best deferred until the data from clinical trials with the pegylated interferons and lamivudine–adefovir combination therapy are available. For patients with advancing fibrosis who are at risk of developing cirrhosis, the options include long-term interferon therapy or prolonged lamivudine monotherapy. At present, we use lamivudine monotherapy in such cases, but patients should be aware that the development of lamivudine resistance may make 'rescue transplantation' impossible. (It should be noted that long term therapy with lamivudine may reverse fibrous lesions including cirrhosis.)

Further reading

Brook MG, McDonald JA, Karayiannis P, *et al*. Randomized controlled trial of interferon alfa 2A (rbe) (Roferon-A) for the treatment of chronic hepatitis B virus (HBV) infection: factors that influence response. *Gut* 1989; **30**: 1116–22.

Dienstag JL, Schiff ER, Wright TL, *et al*. Lamivudine as initial treatment for chronic hepatitis B in the United States. *N Engl J Med* 1999; **341**: 1256–63.

Papatheodoridis GV, Hadziyannis SJ. Diagnosis and management of pre-core

mutant chronic hepatitis B. *J Viral Hep* 2001; **8**: 311–21.

Liaw YF. Treatment of chronic hepatitis B virus infection: who, when, what for and how. *J Gastroenterol Hepatol* 2000; **15(suppl)**: E31–E33.

Questions

1. In patients with chronic hepatitis B who are receiving interferon therapy:
    A. An increase in the serum transaminase level indicates that therapy is not working
    B. Treatment should be given for at least 1 year
    C. The platelet count may decrease
    D. Cirrhosis may deteriorate
    E. Anaemia is a common complication

2. Lamivudine therapy for chronic hepatitis B:
    A. Is given by injection
    B. Leads to seroconversion in 75% of patients after 1 year
    C. May induce mutations in the polymerase protein
    D. May synergize with interferon
    E. Is best given during the immunoactive phase

3. HBeAg-negative chronic hepatitis B:
    A. Is always benign

B. Should be treated with 3 months of interferon
C. Can be diagnosed by sequencing the viral genome
D. May be associated with an increase in the IgM anti HBeAg titre
E. Is always resistant to lamivudine

4. Therapy for chronic hepatitis B:
   A. Should be given when the disease is quiescent
   B. May be most effective when the liver function tests are abnormal
   C. Always requires multiple drugs
   D. May cause a transient increase in the severity of the hepatitis
   E. May generate lamivudine-resistant mutants

Answers

Question 1

A. False – an increase in the serum transaminases often indicates that an immune response is developing that may lead to a seroconversion

B. False – 3 months is adequate
C. True
D. True
E. False

Question 2

A. False – it is an oral therapy
B. False
C. True
D. False
E. True

Question 3

A. False
B. False
C. False
D. True
E. False

Question 4

A. False
B. True
C. False
D. True
E. True

Combined infections

6

Simultaneous infection with more than one virus is unusual, probably because the host defences are activated by the first virus and are then primed and ready to prevent further infections. As discussed in Chapter 1, hepatotropic viruses are able to avoid the host defence systems and this allows infection with multiple different viruses. Even so, patients with more than one infection are uncommon and, in general, the presence of more than one pathogen accelerates disease progression.

Hepatitis delta virus

The hepatitis delta virus is a unique human pathogen that needs the hepatitis B virus to infect cells and cause disease. Hepatitis delta virus is unable to cause infection on its own because it lacks an envelope protein, and the virus requires the surface antigen of the hepatitis B virus in order to propagate itself.

The virus and its replication

The hepatitis delta virus consists of a circular RNA genome that encodes a single protein, the delta antigen. The virus replicates in an unusual fashion that is similar to the process used by plant viroids. The viral RNA is duplicated in a 'rolling circle' mechanism in which antigenomic RNA is produced in a long chain; the long chain of multiple, joined viral genomes is then cleaved by a ribozyme. Ribozymes are enzymes that are formed by loops of RNA and are able to process RNA – hence the hepatitis delta virus RNA is able to form loops that cleave the viral RNA during replication. This unusual replication is an attractive target for the development of antiviral drugs but, to date, none that targets the hepatitis delta virus ribozyme has been developed.

The replication of hepatitis delta virus is thought to be regulated by the single protein that it produces, the hepatitis delta antigen. This protein is found in cells in two different forms:

- a small form that enhances viral replication; and
- a large form that inhibits it.

During hepatitis delta virus replication, the viral genome undergoes a specific nucleotide conversion that changes a uridine to a cytosine at position 1015. This conversion changes the termination codon of the small hepatitis delta antigen and allows RNA translation to continue and so produce the large hepatitis delta antigen. Hence, during replication, the virus changes its genome to allow the production of the inhibitory form of hepatitis delta antigen and then regulates its own replication. What controls the switch from the small to the large form of hepatitis delta antigen is unclear.

Once the hepatitis delta virus RNA has duplicated itself, the new RNA is bound to the hepatitis delta antigen and then packaged into viral particles that are surrounded by the envelope protein of the hepatitis B virus. The virus is then released from the cell using unknown exit pathways.

Natural history of hepatitis delta virus infection

Infection with the hepatitis delta virus is unusual and is common in only a few geographical areas, chiefly the Mediterranean area and South America. The virus can infect only those patients who are co-infected with hepatitis B virus, and two patterns of infection occur:

- co-infection, where both viruses are acquired together; and
- superinfection, where a person who already has chronic hepatitis B virus infection acquires hepatitis delta virus.

In co-infection a severe, acute hepatitis develops that may lead to liver failure requiring transplantation. If the patient survives the initial infection, both viruses are usually eliminated and no further therapy is required. Chronic, persistent infection develops in less than 10% of these patients.

Superinfection with hepatitis delta virus also causes an acute hepatitis and, again, acute liver failure may develop, although this is less common. In contrast to co-infection, in which chronic infection is rare, most patients who are superinfected with hepatitis delta virus go on to develop persistent infection (chronic hepatitis delta).

In chronic hepatitis delta virus infection, both hepatitis B virus and hepatitis delta virus persist in the liver. The natural history of this infection is variable and differs in different geographical regions. In Italy and most other countries chronic hepatitis delta virus infection usually causes an aggressive hepatitis that progresses to cirrhosis within a relatively

few years. However, on the Mediterranean island of Rhodes, hepatitis delta virus infection is common and usually leads to a mild disease that progresses very slowly. In South America, outbreaks of infection occur in which large numbers of people are infected. It is not clear whether these differences in transmission and outcome are due to different viral species or whether they are due to genetic differences in the host population.

Diagnosis of hepatitis delta virus infection

The diagnosis of hepatitis delta virus infection is not difficult if the diagnosis is considered – since the infection is rare in most Western countries it is usually not considered and is therefore too often missed.

A high index of suspicion is required to ensure that cases of hepatitis delta superinfection are recognized. The presence of hepatitis delta virus usually suppresses the replication of the hepatitis B virus and therefore patients tend to have circulating HBsAg in their serum but are usually HBeAg-negative, although the absence of HBeAg is by no means essential for the diagnosis. The liver function tests are usually abnormal, and the diagnosis can be confirmed by assays for antibodies against the hepatitis delta antigen (anti-hepatitis delta antibodies). Hence hepatitis delta virus superinfection should always be considered in patients with hepatitis B surface antigenaemia who have abnormal liver function tests.

The diagnosis can be confirmed by detecting antibodies against hepatitis delta virus in the serum, but a more sensitive test is to stain a liver biopsy for the hepatitis delta antigen using immunohistochemical techniques.

Pathology of chronic hepatitis delta virus infection

As described above, patients with chronic hepatitis B virus infection may either be co-infected or superinfected with hepatitis delta virus. Each of these cases, but particularly the latter, is associated with a marked increase in liver cell damage and inflammation especially in the lobules. Hepatitis delta virus is a cytopathic virus, and the liver damage is characterized by marked acidophilic (apoptotic) liver cell damage.

Since this form of liver damage is relatively uncommon in cases of pure hepatitis B virus infection, its presence is an indication for immunohistochemical

staining for hepatitis delta virus. In the outbreaks of hepatitis delta virus infection that are seen in South America, microvesicular fatty change is a striking histological finding. It should be noted that micovesicular fatty change is also a common finding in acute hepatitis caused by hepatitis A virus. 'Sanded' nuclei, which contain finely granular, eosinophilic centres, may be seen in hepatitis delta virus infection and correlate with the presence of the hepatitis delta virus antigen. Similar nuclear changes can also be due to HBcAg.

The diagnosis of hepatitis delta virus infection can be made most quickly and specifically by immunohistochemical staining (Figs 6.1 and 6.2). There is nuclear staining with or without cytoplasmic staining. The presence of hepatitis delta virus antigen in the liver is, in fact, the gold standard for diagnosing this infection. Unfortunately, at the present time, there is no good, commercially available antibody to the hepatitis delta antigen. In liver transplant patients, hepatitis delta virus antigen can be demonstrated in the absence of hepatitis B. The associated liver damage in these circumstances is very mild.

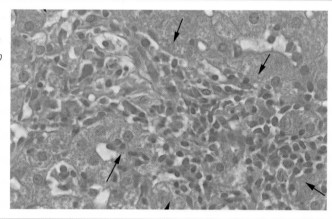

Figure 6.1
Liver biopsy from a patient with chronic HBV who developed a flare up of his disease due to superinfection with HDV. Histologically this was characterised by active lobular inflammation.

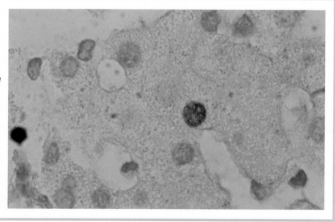

Figure 6.2
Same liver biopsy as in 6.1 stained with an antibody to HDV. The positive nuclear staining illustrated is sensitive and specific confirmation of active infection by HDV.

Management of chronic hepatitis delta virus infection

Although there is no vaccine against hepatitis delta virus itself, the virus depends on the presence of hepatitis B virus for its replication; therefore preventing infection with hepatitis B also protects against the hepatitis delta agent. Hence contacts and partners of patients with chronic hepatitis delta should be vaccinated against hepatitis B.

Table 6.1
A typical liver biopsy report from a patient with hepatitis B virus infection and superimposed hepatitis delta virus infection

---

Macroscopic appearance
A core of brown tissue 2.9 cm in length

Microscopic appearance
Liver with widespread fibrous expansion of portal tracts
There is mild portal inflammation and interface hepatitis but there is marked lobular
inflammation with prominent acidophilic degeneration of hepatocytes
The bile ducts are normal
No ground glass cells are present
Special stains for iron, alpha-1-anti-trypsin bodies and copper-associated protein are
negative
There is no dysplasia

Immunohistochemical staining
5% of cells show nuclear ± cytoplasmic staining for delta antigen
There is focal cytoplasmic staining for HBsAg; staining for HBcAg is negative

Conclusion
An active chronic hepatitis due to hepatitis delta virus infection in a patient with
hepatitis B

Modified HAI score
Grade – 1+0+3+1=5/18
Stage = 2/6

A typical liver biopsy report from a patient with hepatitis B virus infection and superimposed hepatitis delta virus infection is show in Table 6.1.

Patients infected with hepatitis delta virus are at high risk of developing progressive liver disease. It is therefore unfortunate that there is at present no proven, effective therapy for patients with this disease. Short courses of interferon have been tried in patients with chronic hepatitis delta but they are usually unsuccessful. Prolonging the therapy for many months may be of some small benefit and, at present, this appears to be the most effective therapeutic approach. The optimum dose and duration of therapy have not yet been determined and it is likely that the new pegylated interferons will be beneficial in this setting, although clinical trials to confirm this have not yet been completed. Lamivudine therapy has no effect on the hepatitis delta virus but may reduce the liver damage associated with the hepatitis B virus.

For the clinician faced with a patient who has progressive liver disease due to hepatitis delta virus co-infection, there is no consensus on the most appropriate management. Our current approach is to adopt a 'suck it and see' policy that involves trials of antiviral agents with frequent liver biopsies to assess response. We initially use lamivudine for a few months and then perform a biopsy to assess progression. In those patients who appear to improve on this regime, we continue lamivudine monotherapy and monitor liver damage with repeat liver biopsies. For those who do not improve, we commence interferon at a dose of 6–9 Miu three times a week and, again, monitor progress by serial biopsies. It is to be hoped that future clinical trials will determine the most effective therapeutic approach.

Co-infection with other viruses

Co-infection, either with several hepatotropic viruses or with a hepatotropic virus and HIV, is fortunately rare; however, when it does occur interactions between the different viruses alter both the natural history of the disease and the treatment.

Co-infection with hepatitis B virus and hepatitis C virus

Since these two viruses are both blood-borne pathogens, it would be expected that co-infection should be quite common. However, this does not appear to be the case, and co-infection is much less prevalent than predicted. When co-infection is found, it is usually associated with a rapidly progressive disease that leads to cirrhosis within a few years.

The presence of both hepatitis B virus and hepatitis C virus usually leads to inhibition of the replication of one of them. Thus, patients tend to have high levels of hepatitis C viraemia with low levels of hepatitis B virus DNA and undetectable HBeAg, or they tend to be HBeAg-positive with high levels of hepatitis B virus DNA and low levels of hepatitis C virus RNA. In some patients the dominant virus may change with time, and such patients may therefore have dominant hepatitis B on one occasion and dominant hepatitis C on another.

Co-infection with hepatitis B and hepatitis C is very difficult to treat. Standard therapeutic regimes of interferon–ribavirin or lamivudine are rarely successful. Logically these patients should benefit from therapy with interferon plus ribavirin plus lamivudine, but the safety and efficacy of this approach has never been tested and further clinical studies are urgently required in this group of patients.

Although co-infection with hepatitis B virus and hepatitis C virus is uncommon, a number of patients with active hepatitis C have evidence of past exposure to hepatitis B virus (i.e. they have antibodies against the viral proteins, such as anti-hepatitis B virus core antibodies). It is becoming clear that these patients tend to have a diminished response to therapy for their chronic hepatitis C, although the reasons for this are not yet clear.

Co-infection with HIV and hepatitis C virus

In the past, co-infection with HIV and hepatitis C virus was of little hepatological importance as, sadly, patients died of HIV-related immunosuppression long before liver damage developed. Effective antiretroviral therapy has led to a reappraisal of the significance of co-infection and it is now clear that infection with HIV and hepatitis C virus leads to an increase in the severity of both infections. Hence the natural history of chronic hepatitis C virus infection is accelerated and progression to cirrhosis is both more rapid and more common than in patients who are not infected with HIV. This increase in the severity of liver disease in co-infected patients has led to liver disease becoming one of the most common causes of death in HIV-positive patients in the USA.

In addition to the deleterious effects of HIV on hepatitis C, it is now believed that hepatitis C may accelerate the progression of HIV infection and co-infected patients have evidence of more significant lymphocyte functional abnormalities than patients who are infected only with HIV. Thus co-infection with both hepatitis C and HIV accelerates the progression of both viral infections.

Treatment of patients with HIV–hepatitis C co-infection is problematic and few satisfactory studies have been completed. Therapy for HIV must take precedence and patients should be stabilized on an appropriate regime of antiretroviral agents before evaluating the therapeutic options for hepatitis C. Once the patient is stable on antiretroviral therapy, the extent of the liver disease should be determined by a liver biopsy and a decision as to whether to proceed with therapy for hepatitis C discussed. If the liver biopsy indicates severe fibrosis then treatment for hepatitis C virus infection should be recommended using standard regimes of an interferon (preferably a pegylated interferon) and ribavirin.

In patients with dual infections, therapy for HIV is likely to involve a large array of antiretroviral medication. Adding the rigours of interferon therapy with ribavirin to this complex regime often hinders compliance; before embarking upon therapy for hepatitis C, it is important to discuss compliance with the patient and ensure that the patient is willing to take additional medication. Recent increases in our understanding of the natural history of HIV infection have suggested that some patients who are infected with HIV may have stable disease for many years. In such patients it may be appropriate to delay antiretroviral therapy and it may be wise to consider therapy for hepatitis C at this stage (i.e. before highly active antiretroviral therapy is introduced). However, at present there are no clinical trial data to determine whether such an approach is appropriate.

Problems during combination therapy for HIV infection and hepatitis C

The addition of interferon and ribavirin to complex highly active antiretroviral therapy regimes markedly increases the possibility of drug interactions. Although many of the postulated interactions between antiretroviral drugs and ribavirin are theoretical rather than real, the possibility of harmful interactions should be borne in mind.

The most common problem is bone marrow toxicity, and regular assessment of the haemoglobin and white cell count is essential for patients receiving combination therapy. We routinely monitor patients weekly for the first 3 months of therapy and then reduce the frequency of monitoring if the patient's condition is stable.

Co-infection with HIV and hepatitis B virus

Careful consideration of the natural history of chronic hepatitis B and the role of the immune system in the pathogenesis of this disease enables the likely effects of concomitant HIV infection to be predicted. During the immunotolerant phase of chronic hepatitis B virus infection, when high-level viraemia is associated with a minimal immune response, co-infection with HIV usually has little impact. However, if the HIV-related immunosuppression is severe then the level of hepatitis B viraemia may rise markedly and fibrosing cholestatic hepatitis may develop, although this is rare (see page 86).

For patients with the immunoactive form of chronic hepatitis B (high level hepatitis B viraemia with an inflammatory response and marked liver damage), significant HIV infection may reduce the liver inflammation. As the immune response is impaired by HIV infection, the immune-mediated liver damage tends to subside.

During the immunosurveillance phase of chronic hepatitis B virus infection (HBsAg-positive, HBeAg-negative serology with low-level viraemia), immunosuppression due to HIV infection may lead to a reverse seroconversion. The reduction in the immune response against hepatitis B virus may lead to a reactivation of the disease and emergence of detectable levels of HBeAg. If the immune response is restored by antiretroviral therapy, the hepatic infection may be brought under control once again – initially the immune response leads to an increase in liver damage but eventually the immune response may lead to the elimination of the HBeAg once again.

Hence co-infection with HIV may significantly modify the effects of the hepatitis B virus, and careful monitoring of both viruses is required to determine the likely cause of the liver disease.

It is important to be aware of the hepatotoxic effects of the widely used antiretroviral drugs – in patients with HIV infection and hepatitis B virus infection, any change in the liver function tests should be fully investigated, and increases in hepatic inflammation should not be ascribed to activation of the hepatitis B unless other possible causes have been excluded; in general marked changes in liver function tests should be investigated by a liver biopsy in these patients. Immunochemistry is very valuable in assessing liver biopsies from this group of patients.

Management of co-infection with hepatitis B virus and HIV

Interferon therapy has been tried in co-infected patients but there are few reports of success and the benefits of the new pegylated interferons in this group of patients are unclear. For patients with active hepatitis B and HIV co-infection, lamivudine is a logical therapeutic choice because it inhibits the replication of both viruses. However, it is important to be aware of the different doses used in the treatment of these infections – patients with HIV infection require high-dose lamivudine whereas patients with chronic hepatitis B virus infection are usually treated with much lower doses. Close collaboration between the hepatologist and the infectious disease physician is required to ensure that these patients are managed appropriately. It is easy to forget the hepatitis B component of the illness when considering drug changes for the HIV infection, and in co-infected patients the lamivudine therapy should not be stopped even if it is no longer required for suppression of HIV replication.

Further reading

Bonino F, Negro F, Brunetto MR, Verme G. Hepatitis delta virus infection. *Prog Liver Dis* 1990; **9**: 485–96.

Greub G, Ledergerber B, Battegay M, *et al.* Clinical progression, survival, and immune recovery during antiretroviral therapy in patients with HIV-1 and hepatitis C virus coinfection: the Swiss HIV Cohort Study. *Lancet* 2000; **356**: 1800–5

Mathurin P, Thibault V, Kadidja K, *et al.* Replication status and histological features of patients with triple (B, C, D) and dual (B, C) hepatic infections. *J Viral Hep* 2000; **7**: 15–22.

Taylor J. Hepatitis delta virus. *Intervirology* 1999; **42**: 173–8.

Villari D, Raimondo G, Smedile V, *et al.* Hepatitis B-DNA replication and histological patterns in liver biopsy specimens of chronic HBsAg positive patients with and without hepatitis delta virus superinfection. *J Clin Pathol* 1989; **42**: 689–93.

Questions

1. The diagnosis of hepatitis delta:
   A. Should be considered in intravenous drug users
   B. Can only be made in patients who are also infected with hepatitis C
   C. Can be excluded if HBeAg is detected
   D. Is often made in people of Italian descent
   E. Requires immunostaining of a liver biospy

2. Co-infection with hepatitis B virus and hepatitis C virus:
   A. Is very common
   B. Responds well to therapy with interferon and ribavirin
   C. May be associated with HBeAg-negative disease
   D. Causes rapidly progressive liver disease

E. May reduce the effects of
lamivudine on the replication of
hepatitis B virus

3. In co-infection with HIV and hepatitis
C virus:
   A. The hepatitis C virus infection may
   respond to therapy with interferon
   and ribavirin
   B. The HIV infection may progress
   more rapidly
   C. Therapy for HIV should be withheld
   D. Abnormal liver function tests
   always indicate active hepatitis C
   E. Drug interactions are common

4. In co-infection with HIV and hepatitis
B virus:
   A. The HBeAg level may fluctuate
   B. Low-dose lamivudine should be used
   C. The HIV infection progresses at the
   same rate as in patients uninfected
   by hepatitis B virus
   D. HIV protease inhibitors may inhibit
   the replication of hepatitis B virus
   E. Fibrosing cholestatic hepatitis may
   occur

Answers

Question 1

A. True
B. False – the association is with hepatitis B

C. False – it is rarely associated with
HBeAg positivity
D. True
E. False – this is the most sensitive
diagnostic technique but the diagnosis
can be made serologically

Question 2

A. False
B. False
C. True
D. True
E. False

Question 3

A. True
B. True
C. False
D. False – other causes must be
considered
E. True

Question 4

A. True
B. False – high doses are required to treat
the HIV infection
C. True
D. False
E. True

Non-hepatic manifestations

7

The hepatotropic viruses predominantly infect hepatocytes, and the diseases that they cause are primarily hepatological disorders. However, in addition to causing liver damage, these viruses may induce non-hepatic diseases that may require therapy in their own right.

Non-specific extrahepatic manifestations of chronic viral hepatitis

Infection with the hepatitis B virus is remarkably well tolerated and the majority of chronically infected patients are truly asymptomatic unless the complications of cirrhosis develop.

However, this is not the case for patients chronically infected with the hepatitis C virus – these patients have a high incidence of psychiatric disease and, in quality of life studies, patients with chronic hepatitis C virus infection have clear evidence of impaired health related quality of life.

Chronic hepatitis C is common in patients who abuse drugs. Many people who misuse drugs have ongoing psychiatric disease, and it is therefore not surprising to find that a large proportion of patients with chronic hepatitis C also suffer from psychiatric disorders, particularly depression. For many of these patients the onset of the psychiatric disorder predates the onset of the hepatitis and it is clear that these disorders are not causally linked to the viral infection.

> It is important to recognize concurrent psychiatric disease in patients with chronic hepatitis C, since it may respond to treatment with conventional psychiatric medication but is unlikely to improve with antiviral therapy.

Patients with psychiatric problems and hepatitis C should be reviewed by a psychiatrist and should receive appropriate medication for their psychiatric disorder.

A large proportion of patients with chronic hepatitis C virus infection complain of a variety of non-specific symptoms that are not directly attributable to their liver disease and that are not related to pre-existing psychiatric disease. These symptoms include:

- profound fatigue with non-refreshing sleep;
- generalized aches and pains in all limbs;
- flitting arthralgia;
- difficulty in concentrating;
- complaints of short-term memory loss.

More rarely patients complain of crampy abdominal pains and urinary frequency, often associated with right hypochondrial discomfort that waxes and wanes. Taken together, these non-specific symptoms are profoundly debilitating and contribute to the significant impairment in quality of life assessments seen in these patients. The non-specific symptoms associated with chronic hepatitis C virus infection are not related to the severity of the liver disease and are found in patients who have never used drugs as well as in those who are addicted to illicit drugs. The cause of the symptoms is not clear but eradication of the virus leads to a significant improvement; in patients who are disabled by these non-hepatological manifestations, therapy should be considered even if the liver biopsy shows no evidence of significant damage.

Specific extrahepatic manifestations associated with chronic hepatitis C virus infection

Chronic hepatitis C virus infection is common and is usually diagnosed by healthcare professionals. In the past, the virus was passed on during blood transfusions and it is therefore not surprising to find that a very large number of diseases have been found to be associated with chronic hepatitis C virus infection. In the case of many of these diseases it is not clear whether the virus causes the disease or whether the association is purely coincidental. Many of the reported 'associations' are probably mere coincidence.

Mixed essential cryoglobulinaemia

Cryoglobulins are circulating proteins that precipitate out in the cold. They are identified in serum as a precipitate that appears on cooling and dissolves on rewarming. Their detection requires careful planning and preparation – the blood specimen must be kept at 37°C until the blood clots; this involves placing the blood sample into a 37°C water bath immediately after it has been taken. The serum is centrifuged and then kept at 4°C for several days. If cryoglobulins are present a precipitate will form in the cold and the amount of precipitate – the cryocrit – can then be determined. The cryocrit is usually more than 3% in patients with clinical disease.

In chronic hepatitis C the cryoprecipitate usually contains hepatitis C virus RNA as well as immunoglobulins, including a rheumatoid factor, and it is characterized as 'mixed essential cryoglobulin'.

In some regions (such as Italy) chronic hepatitis C is often associated with cryoglobulinaemia, but in other areas (such as the United Kingdom) the virus rarely induces cryoglobulins. In Italy some 36–45% of patients with chronic hepatitis C have circulating cryoglobulins that can be detected by appropriate assays. In most patients the cryoglobulinaemia is silent and causes no disease or symptoms. However, in about 10% of patients with detectable cryoglobulins there is an associated vasculitis with a rash on the limbs, arthralgia, neuropathy and weakness. Typically the rash is episodic and occurs in crops that affect predominantly the lower limbs. The associated neuropathy may induce disabling pain. There may be an associated glomerulonephritis (see next section). The coexisting liver disease is usually mild.

It is not known why some patients develop a cryoglobulinaemia and why only some of these develop clinical symptoms. No correlation with viral genotype, titre or clinical features has been found.

Therapy for mixed essential cryoglobulin involves treating the underlying hepatitis C with interferon and ribavirin. If the virus is eliminated the cryoglobulins disappear, confirming that they are caused by the hepatitis C virus infection. Nearly all patients with hepatitis C-related cryoglobulinaemia respond while on therapy (i.e. the symptoms disappear and the cryocrit is reduced). However when therapy is stopped any relapse and recurrence of viraemia is associated with recurrence of the symptoms and signs of the cryoglobulinaemia. In these patients who have not eliminated the virus after a standard course of therapy it may be appropriate to start antiviral therapy again, and many groups treat such patients with low-dose interferon for many months or even years. This unorthodox approach has never been evaluated in controlled clinical trials but a large number of case reports supports it, and we routinely treat our patients with disabling cryoglobulinaemia in this way.

Glomerulonephritis

Glomerulonephritis is common in patients with chronic hepatitis C virus infection and cryoglobulinaemia – it rarely occurs in the absence of cryoglobulinaemia. The glomerulonephritis may cause either a nephrotic picture or a nephritic picture, and the underlying renal histology may be either a membranous glomerulonephritis or a membranoproliferative glomerulonephritis.

Therapy should be directed at the underlying infection and the patient should be treated with standard combination therapy, provided that the renal function is adequate. If the virus is eradicated the glomerular lesions resolve. There is no information as to whether patients without associated cryoglobulinaemia in whom therapy fails benefit from prolonged interferon therapy.

Porphyria cutanea tarda

Porpyria cutanea tarda is an unusual skin disorder associated with skin fragility and a chronic and recurrent vesicular rash on those parts of the body exposed to the sun, especially the back of the hands. There are sporadic and familial forms of this condition, although both forms may be associated with an underlying metabolic defect (i.e. a deficiency of uroporphryinogen decarboxylase). Cofactors for the development of porphyria cutanea tarda are alcohol and iron overload.

Hepatitis C virus infection is associated with porphyria cutanea tarda in between 8 and 91% of cases, depending on the population surveyed. In our patients it is extremely rare. The role of hepatitis C in the pathogenesis of the skin lesions is unclear and it has been suggested that underlying liver damage, which is usually significant, unmasks the disease in genetically predisposed patients.

The therapy for porphyria cutanea tarda is to remove excess iron by venesection and to eradicate the hepatitis C virus infection with standard therapies.

Autoimmune thyroiditis

Thyroid dysfunction is common in patients with chronic hepatitis C virus infection. The mechanism remains obscure but both hyperthyroidism and hypothyoidism have been reported. The commonest association is with Hashimoto's autoimmune thyroiditis, and patients often have anti-thyroid antibodies (typically anti-TPO antibodies). Thyroid disturbance is more common in women

with hepatitis C and is often associated with a strong family history of thyroid disease.

All patients with chronic hepatitis C virus infection should have their thyroid function tested on at least one occasion and it is wise to assess anti-thyroid antibodies since high titres of anti-TPO antibodies have been associated with the later development of thyroid dysfunction.

A particular problem in patients with hepatitis C virus infection is the development of thyroid disease during interferon therapy. The fatigue related to hypothyroidism is easily misdiagnosed as a side effect of therapy and, unless thyroid disease is considered and specifically tested for, the condition is easily missed. Encouraging patients to 'put up with the side effects of interferon' when they are developing hypothyroidism does little to enhance the doctor–patient relationship. Although thyroid dysfunction is more common in patients who have high titres of anti-thyroid antibodies before therapy, the condition can develop *de novo* during therapy; we recommend that all patients receiving interferon have regular thyroid function tests.

Patients with chronic hepatitis C who develop thyroid disease should receive appropriate hormonal therapy – and the advice of an experienced endocrinologist should be sought. Although interferon may induce the development of thyroid disease, withdrawal of the interferon does not lead to a reversal of the thyroid dysfunction and therefore antiviral therapy should be continued if thyroid disease develops.

B cell lymphoma

B cell lymphoma (non-Hodgkins B cell lymphoma) is a rare malignancy that has been associated with chronic hepatitis C virus infection. The disorder seems to be particularly prevalent in patients with hepatitis C-related cryoglobulinaemia but it is not yet known whether prolonged interferon therapy for the cryoglobulinaemia reduces the risk of lymphoma – although it is generally assumed that viral eradication does reduce the risk of subsequent lymphoma, this has not been formally proven.

Skin disorders

A number of dermatological disorders have been reported to be associated with chronic hepatitis C virus infection. The most common of these is lichen planus. This irritating disorder may improve with successful therapy for the hepatitis C

virus infection, but in many patients therapy for the viral infection does not improve the skin disorder; in some patients therapy may exacerbate it.

A rare complication of chronic hepatitis C virus infection is pyoderma gangrenosum, which may occur in the absence of cryoglobulins and normally improves if the virus is eradicated.

Specific extrahepatic manifestations of hepatitis B virus infection

The majority of the extrahepatic manifestations associated with hepatitis B viral infection are related to the magnitude of the antiviral immune response, and most of the non-hepatic diseases are related to antigen–antibody deposition. All of these diseases are extremely rare and affect only a tiny proportion of patients infected with the hepatitis B virus.

Serum sickness-like syndromes

This very rare syndrome is seen in acute hepatitis B virus infection, where it precedes the development of the hepatitis, and in the early stages of chronic hepatitis. It is characterized by fever, skin rashes and arthralgia. In acute disease the symptoms usually improve before the onset of jaundice. The syndrome is usually benign and no therapy is required.

Polyarteritis nodosa

Polyarteritis nodosa is a rare disorder in which a vasculitis develops that involves medium-sized arteries in multiple organ systems. It is characterized by hypertension, renal failure, asthma and ischaemia (including stroke, intestinal ischaemia, acalulous cholecystitis and mononeuritis multiplex). Although the clinical course is very variable, the mortality rate is high. Between 10 and 50% of patients with polyarteritis nodosa have HBsAg in their serum and most also have circulating HBeAg. As is the case with the serum sickness-like syndromes described above, this condition is more common in the early stages of chronic hepatitis B. The disease is probably the result of deposition of circulating immune complexes in the walls of the involved blood vessels. Although polyarteritis is an uncommon complication of chronic hepatitis B, it is seen more frequently in certain ethnic groups (e.g. Inuit), which suggests that host genetic factors may be involved in pathogenesis.

In the early stages of the illness,

immunosuppressive therapy is more important than treating the underlying chronic hepatitis B virus infection, and the polyarteritis should be treated with high doses of corticosteroids and cyclophosphamide. If the patient clears the hepatitis B virus infection (i.e. eliminates the HBsAg) the associated polyarteritis nodosa usually resolves. It is possible that therapy with lamivudine may improve the vasculitis associated with chronic hepatitis B, but no studies have yet been performed to examine this.

Glomerulonephritis

Glomerulonephritis associated with hepatitis B virus infection commonly occurs in children and usually presents as the nephrotic syndrome. Renal biopsy usually shows membranous glomerulonephritis and the renal disease often resolves spontaneously (between 30 and 60% of children have spontaneous resolution of their renal disease). This resolution is often associated with seroconversion from HBeAg positivity to HBeAb positivity, and this seroconversion may be induced by treatment with interferon. No studies with lamivudine have yet been reported in this group of patients.

In adults, the renal disease is more

frequently progressive and response to interferon is uncommon. Renal biopsy shows either a membranous glomerulonephritis (the most common finding) or a membranoproliferative glomerulonephritis. The latter is more likely to be associated with progressive renal disease. As is the case with polyarteritis nodosa, the pathogenesis of the glomerulonephritis is thought to be due to the deposition of circulating immune complexes, although it is possible that the complexes may be formed *in situ*. The immune complexes can be visualized on electron microscopy within the capillary basement membrane and HBsAg or HBeAg (or both) can be demonstrated immunohistochemically. Again one would predict that these patients would benefit from lamivudine therapy but no cases have yet been described in which this treatment has been used.

Other non-hepatic manifestations of chronic hepatitis B virus infection

A number of different skin rashes have been described in association with hepatitis B virus infection. These include hives and a fleeting maculopapular rash (which are seen mainly in adult women early in the course of chronic hepatitis B virus infection), and an acropapular dermatitis (Gianotti's syndrome) in children, especially in acute infection. Gianotti's syndrome is characterized by a transient, episodic, itchy, erythematous and palpable rash, usually on the arms and legs. It may leave a residual discoloration of the skin.

Arthralgia may be associated with chronic hepatitis B and is said to be more common in adult women. The small joints of the hands and the joints of the wrists, hips and knees are most frequently involved. The arthralgia is migratory and a fully developed arthritis is extremely rare.

In our experience arthralgia in association with hepatitis B is rare but the complaint is common in patients with chronic hepatitis C. It is not clear whether previous reports of arthralgia associated with chronic hepatitis B were in fact seen in patients with chronic hepatitis C whose second virus was not identified.

Further reading

Hadziyannis S. Non hepatic manifestations of chronic HCV infection. *J Viral Hep* 1997; **4**: 1–17.

Forton D, Allsop J, Main J, Foster G, Thomas H, Taylor-Robinson S. Evidence for a cerebral effect of the hepatitis C virus. *Lancet* 2001; **358**: 38–9.

Foster GR, Goldin RD, Thomas HC, Chronic hepatitis C virus infection causes a significant reduction in quality of life in the absence of cirrhosis. *Hepatology* 1998; **27**: 209–13.

Questions

1. Chronic fatigue in patients with chronic hepatitis C:
   A. Usually improves if the virus is eradicated
   B. May be due to thyroid disease
   C. Is related to the severity of the liver disease
   D. May be due to haemolytic anaemia
   E. May be a justification for therapy

2. The following skin diseases may complicate chronic viral hepatitis:
   A. Eczema
   B. Lichen planus
   C. Dermatitis herpetiformis
   D. Porphyria cutanea tarda
   E. Pyoderma gangrenosum

3. Hepatitis C-associated cryoglobulinaemia:
   A. Is always benign
   B. Is common in Afro-Caribbeans
   C. May be associated with glomerulonephritis
   D. May cause peripheral neuropathy
   E. May be treated with long-term interferon

4. Renal disease associated with chronic hepatitis B virus infection:
   A. May deteriorate with interferon therapy
   B. Is more common in children
   C. May cause a nephrotic syndrome
   D. Has a poor prognosis
   E. Is associated with cryoglobulinaemia

Answers

Question 1

A. True
B. True
C. False
D. False
E. True

Question 2

A. False
B. True
C. False
D. True
E. True

Question 3

A. False
B. False
C. True
D. True
E. True

Question 4

A. False
B. True
C. True
D. False
E. False

Difficult-to-treat patient groups

8

A number of patient groups pose particular management problems. Inevitably such patients are uncommon and, in general, have been excluded from clinical trials. Therapy for such patients is often opinion-based rather than evidence-based.

Cirrhosis

Cirrhosis is defined as 'irreversible fibrosis of the liver' and is characterized histologically by the presence of circles of collagen. Recent data have challenged the view that cirrhosis is irreversible, and studies from patients with cirrhosis caused by both HCV and HBV have suggested that, if the virus can be eliminated, the fibrosis may regress and the liver may then return to a 'precirrhotic' state. This important finding requires further confirmation.

Patients with histologically proven cirrhosis can be divided into:

- those with well-compensated cirrhosis; and
- those with decompensated cirrhosis.

In essence patients with well-compensated cirrhosis have normal hepatic synthetic function (normal serum albumin, clotting factors and bilirubin) with no evidence of portal hypertension whereas patients with decompensated cirrhosis have signs of impaired hepatic function as well as features of portal hypertension. The extent of hepatic impairment is usually assessed by reference to the Childs–Pugh score. This is a scoring system that assesses the severity of the cirrhotic change. It has been widely used in clinical trials and may be useful in clinical practice since it allows the extent of the hepatic disease to be assessed. Table 8.1 shows the salient features of this scoring system.

All patients with cirrhosis should be evaluated for the presence of oesophageal varices (usually by endoscopy) and, if varices are found, primary prophylaxis with propranolol should be commenced and beta-blockers should be given at a dose that reduces the resting pulse rate by 30%. These patients should be considered for entry into ultrasound screening programmes (see page 150).

Management of hepatitis C-related cirrhosis

Patients with cirrhosis induced by chronic hepatitis C do respond to therapy, albeit at a lower rate than patients with lesser degrees of fibrosis. Follow-up studies comparing treated and untreated patients suggest that the rate of development of decompensated disease and the development of liver cell cancer may be reduced in patients who have received interferon therapy. This benefit is most marked in patients who have cleared the virus, but even patients who have not responded to therapy by eliminating the virus may have a reduced rate of complications.

These studies indicate that patients with hepatitis C-related cirrhosis may derive considerable benefit from therapy, but the optimum regime is not yet clear. Interferon monotherapy eradicates the virus in very few patients but it may significantly reduce the rate of development of primary liver cancer. The 40 kD pegylated interferon has been assessed as monotherapy in a clinical trial involving only patients with advanced fibrosis or cirrhosis; 30% of those receiving therapy were cured. It seems likely that the addition of ribavirin to a pegylated interferon will improve response rates further, and this is probably the optimum therapy for these patients.

Table 8.1
The Childs–Pugh score

Points scored	Encephalopathy grade*	Bilirubin (μmol/l)	Albumin (g/l)	Prolongation of prothrombin time (seconds)
1	—	<25	>35	1–4
2	I, II	25–40	28–35	4–6
3	III, IV	>40	<28	>6

*Grading of encephalopathy:

Grade I – confused, altered mood or behaviour, psychometric defects.

Grade II – drowsy, inappropriate behaviour

Grade III – stuporous but speaking and obeying simple commands; inarticulate speech, marked confusion

Grade IV – Coma

Grade A is a score of 5–6

Grade B is a score of 7–9

Grade C is a score of 10–15

In addition to its antiviral and immunomodulatory effects, interferon has antifibrotic properties and may reduce hepatic fibrosis. This has led to suggestions that patients with cirrhosis who have not eliminated the virus after a course of pegylated interferon plus ribavirin should receive long-term maintenance therapy to improve the underlying fibrosis. This approach is currently being prospectively studied in the USA, where the 40 kD pegylated interferon (at a dose of 90 μg/week) will be administered for several years to patients with cirrhosis. The outcome of this study is awaited with interest. In the absence of evidence that prolonged interferon therapy is beneficial to patients with hepatitis C-related cirrhosis we do not routinely use this approach, but we continue therapy for at least 6 months in all patients with cirrhosis even if they have not shown a virological response after 3 months of therapy.

Therapy with interferon invariably leads

to a decrease in both the platelet count and the white cell count and, in the presence of hypersplenism, may lead to a dangerous decline in these parameters. In patients with well-compensated cirrhosis who have a platelet count of more than 90×10^9 cells/l and a total white cell count of more than 2.5×10^9 cells/l, this rarely causes significant problems, although dose adjustments may be necessary in some patients. In patients with decompensated cirrhosis who have platelet counts and white cell counts that are lower than these levels, interferon therapy may lead to a dangerous fall in either the platelet count or the white cell count, and these patients should receive therapy only in centres with experience in the management of this difficult patient group.

Patients with hepatitis C who develop decompensated cirrhosis (Childs–Pugh grade C) should be considered for liver transplantation, and local guidelines about suitability for surgery should be consulted and applied.

Liver transplantation for chronic hepatitis C-induced cirrhosis

The management of patients undergoing liver transplantation is complex and is beyond the scope of this book. For patients with chronic hepatitis C who undergo liver transplantation, either for decompensated liver disease or hepatocellular carcinoma, the short-term outlook is very good. As with all patients undergoing transplantation, the risks of surgery are high but over 80% of patients are likely to survive the operation and return home. Unfortunately the hepatitis C virus always infects the new liver and in some patients the disease recurs in an aggressive form. The natural history of hepatitis C after liver transplantation is not yet known but it is becoming clear that there is a significant increase in mortality over the first 10 years. Thus 20% of patients develop cirrhosis within 1 year of transplantation and a small proportion die of hepatitis C-related liver disease within 5 years of transplantation. Among those who survive the first few years, some have persistent viraemia with no significant liver damage and others have severe fibrosis. It seems likely that many patients will develop severe liver disease within 10 years of transplantation.

The factors that determine mild or severe recurrence are under intensive investigation, but it is not yet clear whether increasing the immunosuppression increases or decreases the chances of developing severe recurrence. The optimum therapy for these patients is still unknown, but it is clear that these complex cases should be managed by centres with experience in the management of such patients.

Management of hepatitis B-related cirrhosis

Patients with hepatitis B-related cirrhosis and active disease (i.e. the immunoactive phase or the immunoescape phase) have a high probability of progressing to decompensated cirrhosis or primary liver cell cancer (or both). Successful therapy for these patients may significantly reduce the risks of disease progression but is not without risk.

Interferon therapy

In patients with hepatitis B-related cirrhosis and immunoactive disease (HBeAg-positive disease with high serum transaminase levels and a high necroinflammatory score), interferon therapy may induce seroconversion and reduce the risk of disease progression. However, during the seroconversion hepatitis there is a transient increase in the amount of hepatocyte damage since interferon increases the immunologically mediated liver cell destruction. In patients with impaired hepatic synthetic function this may precipitate liver failure.

Interferon therapy should only be undertaken in patients with hepatitis B-related cirrhosis if the liver function is well preserved and if the patient is willing to undergo transplantation. It is worth discussing the patient with the local transplant centre and obtaining approval for transplantation before therapy is started. Once the safety net of transplantation has been put in place, interferon therapy may be started. If possible, standard doses of non-pegylated interferon should be used (9 Miu three times a week) but the white cell count and platelet count should be monitored weekly along with the serum bilirubin concentration, serum albumin concentration and clotting factors. If there is any deterioration in hepatic synthetic function, therapy should be discontinued and the patient referred for urgent consideration of transplantation.

Lamivudine therapy

In patients who have well-compensated cirrhosis, lamivudine appears to be safe and well tolerated and may be used at normal doses. In patients with hepatitis B-related cirrhosis, lamivudine almost invariably reduces the hepatic inflammation and may improve hepatic synthetic function. Unfortunately lamivudine monotherapy may lead to the development of YMDD mutants, which reduce the efficacy of the drug (see page 98). Since successful hepatic transplantation for patients with hepatitis B requires an effective antiviral agent, the development of lamivudine resistance may preclude transplantation.

Hence lamivudine therapy in patients with advanced liver disease may improve hepatic function but may prevent transplantation. The drug should therefore be used with caution in this setting. In patients who are not suitable for transplantation or who are likely to wait a prolonged time for a suitable organ, the benefits of lamivudine therapy are likely to outweigh the risks, and the drug should probably be used. In patients who have markedly abnormal liver function tests and who are very likely to seroconvert and develop antibodies against HBeAg while receiving lamivudine (i.e. those with serum transaminases levels more than five times the upper limit of normal) the benefits once again outweigh the risks and the drug should be used. On the other hand, patients who are good candidates for transplantation and who have mildly elevated liver function tests are unlikely to respond rapidly to lamivudine therapy, and the chance of a mutant developing and precluding transplantation is high. In these patients it may be wiser to retain lamivudine for the post-transplant period, and we do not use lamivudine in this group of patients. Once alternative

nucleoside analogues that are active against the lamivudine-resistant mutants have been developed, it is likely that combination therapy with multiple drugs will become the treatment of choice for patients with hepatitis B-related cirrhosis.

Clearly the use of lamivudine or interferon in patients with hepatitis B-related cirrhosis poses considerable problems and the issues should be discussed with the patient and the local transplant centre before a final decision is reached.

Liver transplantation for patients with hepatitis B-related cirrhosis

In the past, patients with hepatitis B related cirrhosis were considered poor candidates for transplantation since viral recurrence was inevitable and the immunosuppression necessary for successful transplantation invariably led to the rapid development of fibrosis in the new liver. The development of effective antiviral agents has changed this gloomy prognosis and patients with hepatitis B are now regarded as good candidates for transplantation. It is essential that high-level viral replication is avoided after transplantation and this can be achieved by giving intravenous HBIg during the operation and regularly thereafter along with an antiviral agent such as lamivudine. The optimal regime is currently being evaluated, and it is not yet clear how often the HBIg needs to be administered. At present lamivudine is the only reverse transcriptase inhibitor used after transplantation and this has led to the development of resistance in some patients; it is likely that alternative regimens involving multiple drugs will be developed in the near future.

Patients receiving immunosuppressive medication

Patients receiving immunosuppressive medication for coexisting medical problems pose particular management problems. Hepatitis B- and hepatitis C-related disease is often more aggressive in these patients and the currently available treatments are relatively ineffective. Clearly the degree of immunosuppression modifies the disease progression and the likelihood of a response to therapy, and as a general rule the immunosuppressive therapy should be reduced to a minimum in patients with coexisiting viral hepatitis.

Management of immunosuppressed patients with chronic hepatitis C

The natural history of chronic hepatitis C in patients receiving immunosuppressive therapy (e.g. renal transplant patients) has not yet been examined in detail. All of the available evidence suggests that the liver disease is likely to progress at an accelerated rate, but there is enormous patient–patient variability. In some patients the liver disease remains mild for many years despite the presence of quite significant immunosuppression whereas in others the liver disease accelerates and progresses to cirrhosis within a few years. Unfortunately the proportion of patients who develop mild disease or aggressive disease has not yet been determined, and the optimal immunosuppressive regimens have not yet been evaluated.

Interferon is a potent immunostimulator and, when given to patients with autoimmune disorders, it often increases the immunological disease. Thus interferon may exacerbate conditions such as rheumatoid arthritis and systemic lupus erythematosus and it has been shown to induce rejection of renal transplants in 30% of patients. Patients receiving interferon therefore often find that any immunologically mediated disease deteriorates during therapy, necessitating an increase in immunosuppressive medication. Unfortunately interferon therapy for chronic hepatitis C is less effective in the presence of immunosuppressive agents, and during therapy the clinician is often forced to increase the level of immunosuppression and thereby further compromise the effectiveness of the interferon.

It is clear that therapy in this group of patients is extremely difficult and often unsatisfactory. In general, therapy for hepatitis C is best avoided in patients receiving immunosuppressive therapy, and our policy is to monitor such patients with serial liver biopsies. We do not offer therapy to patients with moderate disease and we only consider therapy in those who have advanced fibrosis (grade 5 or 6 on the modified HAI (Ishak) scoring system). In these patients we reduce immunosuppression to the lowest tolerated level and use a standard antiviral therapeutic regimen of an interferon and ribavirin. Patients should be warned that their immunological disease may deteriorate while they are on therapy, and they should be aware that the chances of a virlogical cure are slender.

The position is most difficult in patients who have a functioning renal transplant. If these patients are treated there is a high probability that they will lose their renal transplant and will require dialysis. In our experience most patients with a functioning renal transplant elect not to receive antiviral therapy and to retain the good quality of life that is associated with a functioning renal transplant. The patient's wishes must, of course, be respected.

Management of patients with hepatitis B

The management of patients with chronic hepatitis B virus infection who are receiving immunosuppressive medication is dependent on the level of replication of the virus.

High-level hepatitis B viral replication
In patients with significant immunosuppression who have high-level replication of the hepatitis B virus (i.e. patients in the immunoactive or immunoescape phase), there is a significant risk of the development of fibrosing cholestatic hepatitis (see page 86). This disorder is rapidly fatal but responds well to lamivudine therapy. All patients with fibrosing cholestatic hepatitis should be treated with lamivudine as a matter of course. A small proportion will develop lamivudine-resistant mutations that will lead to treatment failure. In these patients therapy with lamivudine plus adefovir has been reported to induce control of viral replication and improvement in liver histology. The long-term outcome in this setting is not yet clear and whether mutants resistant to lamivudine and

adefovir will eventually emerge and lead to further disease is currently unknown.

In some patients with chronic hepatitis B and ongoing immunosuppressive therapy, the level of viral replication remains below the threshold for the development of fibrosing cholestatic hepatitis, and such patients may 'tolerate' the virus for long periods of time. Appropriate measures should be taken to protect family members from infection, and such patients should be carefully monitored. Disease activation should prompt the introduction of lamivudine therapy. Interferon therapy is of little value in this setting and, in view of the risk of aggravating the underlying autoimmune disease, should be avoided.

Low-level hepatitis B viral replication

Many patients with low-level hepatitis B virus infection who are HBeAg negative with low levels of circulating hepatitis B virus DNA (i.e. patients in the immunosurveillance phase) tolerate immunosuppressive therapy well – the level of viraemia does not alter and no problems are encountered. However, a small proportion of these patients 'reverse seroconvert' when immunosuppressive therapy is introduced. In these patients, the level of viral replication increases markedly and there is a recurrence of active liver disease, which may progress to

fibrosing cholestatic hepatitis. Reactivation of the hepatitis B virus infection has been successfully prevented by prior therapy with lamivudine but the long-term outcome of this approach is unknown, and it is also not yet known whether this approach will lead to the development of lamivudine-resisitant mutants.

The risk factors that influence the development of significant disease with immunosuppressive therapy are unknown and it is therefore impossible to predict which patients will develop disease recurrence. Anecdotal evidence suggests that profound immunosuppression (such as that associated with chemotherapy) and high levels of hepatitis B virus DNA before the initiation of immunosuppressive therapy are often associated with disease recurrence. Our policy is to treat all patients who are HBsAg-positive with lamivudine before chemotherapy and to use lamivudine in patients about to start any immunosuppressive therapy if their hepatitis B virus DNA level is greater than 10^4 copies/ml.

Further reading

Backmund M, Meyer K, Von Zielonka M, Eichenlaub D. Treatment of hepatitis C infection in injection drug users. *Hepatology* 2001; **34**: 188–93.

Hadziyannis SJ, Vassilopoulos D. Complex management issues: management of HCV in the atypical patient. *Ballieres Best Pract Res Clin Gastroenterol* 2000; **14**: 277–91.

Heathcote EJ, Shiffman ML, Cooksley WG, et al. Peginterferon alfa-2a in patients with chronic hepatitis C and cirrhosis. *N Engl J Med* 2000; **343**: 1673–80.

Villeneuve JP, Condreay LD, Willems B, et al. Lamivudine treatment for decompensated cirrhosis resulting from chronic hepatitis B. *Hepatology* 2000; **31**: 207–10.

Questions

1. In patients with hepatitis C-related cirrhosis:
   A. Ribavirin monotherapy may be of value
   B. Interferon therapy may reduce the risk of malignant change
   C. Combination therapy with interferon and ribavirin is of no value
   D. Malignant change may occur in 5% of patients a year
   E. Transplantation is always associated with viral recurrence

2. In patients with hepatitis B-related cirrhosis:
   A. Lamivudine may improve the liver function tests
   B. Interferon therapy may be curative
   C. Malignant change is unusual
   D. Portal hypertension may be exacerbated by lamivudine therapy
   E. The HBeAg is always negative

3. Immunosuppression:
   A. May lead to reverse seroconversion from HBeAg-negative to HBeAg-positive
   B. Is beneficial in patients with chronic hepatitis C
   C. Is an absolute contraindication to ribavirin
   D. May reduce the response rates in patients with chronic hepatitis C
   E. Is always safe in patients who are HBsAg-positive

4. Liver transplantation for patients with viral hepatitis:
   A. Is the commonest indication for transplantation in the USA
   B. Is contraindicated if HBeAg is present
   C. Always requires pretransplant antiviral therapy
   D. May be associated with fibrosing cholestatic hepatitis
   E. Cures hepatitis B and hepatitis C

Answers

Question 1

A. False
B. True
C. False – some 5–10% may respond, but response rates are much higher with the pegylated interferons and ribavirin
D. True
E. True

Question 2

A. True
B. True – but decompensation may occur during therapy
C. False
D. False
E. False

Question 3

A. True
B. False
C. False
D. True
E. False

Question 4

A. True
B. False
C. False
D. True
E. False

Hepatocellular carcinoma

9

Hepatocelluar carcinoma (HCC) is one of the world's most common cancers and it is often associated with chronic viral hepatitis.

All patients with cirrhosis from whatever cause are at risk of liver cell cancer but the risk is particularly high in those with cirrhosis due to viral infection – the risk ranges from 3% per year for Western patients to 6% per year for Japanese patients. Patients with chronic viral hepatitis who do not have cirrhosis have a slightly increased risk of liver cell cancer but the risk is much less than in those with cirrhosis.

Diagnosis of hepatocellular carcinoma

The identification of a primary liver cell cancer arising in a cirrhotic, nodular liver is extremely difficult. Large tumours (more than 4 cm in diameter) are usually easy to identify correctly but, sadly, such lesions are usually untreatable. Small cancers may be treatable and hence their correct identification is a matter of some importance. Correctly distinguishing small, treatable cancers from regenerative liver nodules can be problematic and no single technique is entirely satisfactory.

The correct diagnosis can usually be made only by integrating the information from multiple different approaches; however, even intensive investigation may fail in some cases.

Imaging

Unfortunately there is no one imaging technique that will correctly identify all HCCs, and all of the current techniques have their strengths and weaknesses (Table 9.1 and Fig. 9.1).

Although the sensitivity and specificity of current imaging modalities appear similar in published studies (each modality has a sensitivity of around 80–90%), some tumours are easier to see with one modality than another. Thus we have seen biopsy proven HCC that were invisible to all imaging modalities except ultrasound and we have treated patients when only MRI scanning identified a lesion.

Table 9.1
Advantages and disadvantages of imaging modalities used in the investigation primary liver cell cancers

Modality	Advantages	Disadvantages
Ultrasound	Inexpensive No ionizing radiation Repeatable	Operator dependent
CT scanning	Allows the entire abdomen and chest to be examined for tumour spread Good anatomical localization	Expensive Ionizing radiation
Angiography	Combined with CT scanning may be very sensitive May allow contemporaneous injection of cytotoxic agents directly into the tumour	Ionizing radiation Operator-dependent Involves arterial puncture Expensive
MRI scanning	Allows the entire abdomen and chest to be examined for tumour spread Good anatomical localization No ionizing radiation Repeatable	Expensive Not yet widely available

Figure 9.1
(a) CT scan from a patient with hepatitis C related cirrhosis. Note that a single nodule is seen on this enhanced scan.
(b) Angiogram from the same patient. Note that multiple lesions are now visible. This patient underwent transplantation and the explanted liver showed multiple HCC.

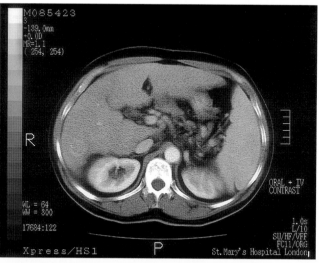

A

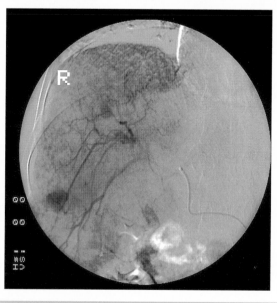

B

In suspicious cases it may be necessary to use multiple imaging techniques to identify the lesion correctly, but even when all modalities are used some lesions will still be missed.

All imaging techniques are, to a greater or lesser extent, operator-dependent and it is important to liaise closely with the radiologist to ensure that local expertise and experience is put to best use.

Ultrasound

Ultrasound is often used as a screening test for HCC in patients with cirrhosis, and it is usually the first form of imaging to be performed in patients suspected of having a tumour. The procedure is relatively inexpensive; moreover it is non-invasive and is not associated with exposure to ionizing radiation. However, the technique is critically dependent on the expertise of the operator and while experienced operators may detect lesions as small as 0.5 cm many ultrasonographers can identify only much larger lesions.

The smallest lesions are hypoechoic but they become hyperechoic with irregular margins as they enlarge. Attempts to improve the sensitivity and specificity of ultrasound have involved intravenous contrast agents (microbubbles). These agents are currently being evaluated but, at present, they seem able to improve the diagnostic accuracy of inexperienced operators, although they may be of less value to experienced hepatic ultrasonographers.

Computed tomography scanning

Computed tomography (CT) scanning is now widely available and, when performed with the administration of contrast, is as sensitive as ultrasound. It has the advantage that more of the body can be examined and a search made for primary or secondary tumours outside the liver. However, the technique is more expensive than ultrasound and exposes the patient to ionizing radiation. Liver cell cancers are seen as hypodense areas that do not enhance with contrast.

Hepatic angiography

Hepatic angiography involves a catheter being inserted into the hepatic artery via the femoral artery and contrast being injected into the liver. The technique may be useful for the evaluation of difficult lesions but it subjects the patient to arterial puncture, contrast administration and ionizing radiation; moreover it is expensive and difficult to perform. Although complications are rare, arterial puncture in patients with advanced liver disease is not without risk and this technique is probably best reserved for cases in which less invasive imaging techniques have not identified a lesion in a patient who is believed to be at high risk.

During hepatic angiography the contrast agent Lipiodol is injected into the hepatic artery; in the past, this oily contrast material was used as a vehicle for the administration of fat soluble cytotoxic agents. This approach had the advantage that a diagnostic procedure could be combined with a therapeutic manoeuvre and led to the widespread use of angiography for the diagnosis of liver cancers. Controlled clinical trials have now shown that intra-arterial administration of current chemotherapeutic agents is not beneficial and this approach has therefore drifted out of fashion. However the direct intra-arterial administration of high concentrations of cytotoxic agents is appealing and, as new agents are developed, it is likely that this approach will once again be evaluated.

When hepatic angiography does not identify a tumour during the initial procedure, a repeat CT scan should be performed 2 weeks later, since the contrast may 'pool' in a tumour that may then be visualized.

Magnetic resonance imaging

Magnetic resonance imaging (MRI) is becoming increasingly popular for the diagnosis of hepatic tumours. Like CT scanning, this technique can examine large areas of the chest and abdomen in a single session, but no ionizing radiation is involved and hence the imaging can be repeated on numerous occasions without undue risk to the patient. The use of intravenous contrast agents significantly increases the sensitivity of the procedure but this also increases the costs. The main drawbacks to MRI are that the machines are expensive and expertise in their use is currently limited.

Biochemical tests

Serum alpha-fetoprotein concentration

Alpha fetoprotein (AFP) is a tumour marker that is produced by approximately 50% of HCCs. Unfortunately the protein is also released by proliferating hepatocytes and hence an increase in the serum concentration is not diagnostic of liver cancer. The test is, however, widely used both as a screening test and to assess the significance of space-occupying lesions. The normal range for serum AFP levels is 0–10 ng/ ml; when the level is over 500 ng/ml, a liver cell cancer is almost certainly present. A few other cancers, such as germ cell tumours of the testes or ovary, may also cause very high serum levels of AFP, but in the context of a patient with cirrhosis due to viral infection, such a high level is almost always caused by an HCC.

AFP levels between 200 and 500 ng/ml may be caused by a number of foregut tumours (including cancer of the pancreas) and hence patients with AFP readings in this range require careful assessment, including detailed imaging of the upper abdomen.

The most common clinical scenario (and the most difficult) is how to investigate a patient with cirrhosis caused by viral liver disease who has a slightly raised serum AFP concentration (50–100 ng/ml). This level is suggestive of malignancy, but such levels may also be seen in patients with cirrhosis who have active liver regeneration. In this setting, serial levels are helpful, since a stable serum AFP concentration is unlikely to be due to cancer whereas a rapidly rising level is probably related to hepatic neoplasia.

In general it is wise to perform at least one imaging investigation in all patients with an elevated serum AFP level. Ultrasound is the most appropriate investigation, because it is easy to repeat; if an ultrasound scan is normal, a follow-up scan should be performed in a few

months' time. If the AFP level is rising rapidly and the ultrasound is normal then further imaging at this stage may be helpful. Our approach to an elevated AFP level is shown in Figure 9.2, but investigations should be tailored to make best use of local facilities and expertise.

In addition to acting as a marker for HCC, the serum AFP level may indicate the probability of a cancer developing. The risk of HCC is much greater in those who have slightly raised serum AFP concentrations, and these patients should be monitored intensively, probably by ultrasound scans every 3 months.

Histology

The major differential diagnosis of a space-occupying lesion in a cirrhotic liver is between:

- macroregenerative nodules (including dysplastic nodules); and
- hepatocellular carcinomas.

For all practical purposes, liver cell adenomas are not seen in cirrhotic livers and this diagnosis should be treated with considerable suspicion.

Macroregenerative nodules and dysplastic nodules are important for two reasons:

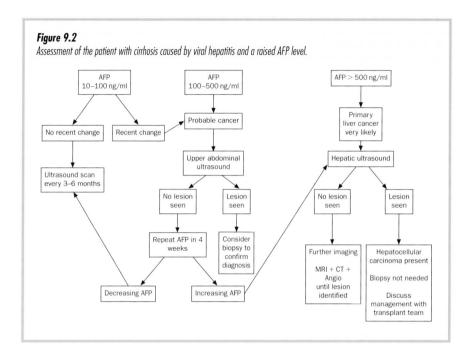

Figure 9.2
Assessment of the patient with cirrhosis caused by viral hepatitis and a raised AFP level.

- they need to be distinguished on imaging and histology from liver cell cancers; and
- they may be premalignant.

Heptocellular carcinoma may arise either within these nodules or it may be seen elsewhere in a liver containing one or more nodules. Neither macroregenerative nodules nor dysplastic nodules are associated with any specific clinical or biochemical features, but serum AFP levels may be raised. Explanted cirrhotic livers should be carefully examined for the presence of all these lesions.

Macroregenerative nodules and dysplastic nodules
These lesions include adenomatous hyperplasia macroregenerative nodules (MRN) types 1 and 2.

Macroscopic appearance
The lesions are over 0.8 cm in diameter, although most are less than 1.5 cm. They may be single or multiple. They are sharply circumscribed and differ from the

surrounding liver in colour (they may be paler or bile-stained) and texture, and they tend to bulge above the cut surface. They are almost always seen in cirrhotic livers and are more common in cases of macronodular cirrhosis than in cases of micronodular cirrhosis.

Microscopic appearance

The liver architecture is relatively preserved and portal tracts may be present. This distinguishes these lesions from liver cell adenomas, although these features may be seen in liver cell carcinomas originating in macroregenerative nodules. The component hepatocytes resemble normal hepatocytes but the liver cell plates are 2–3 cells thick (as is the case in cirrhotic livers). The hepatocytes may contain more or less fat, glycogen and iron than the surrounding liver. They may contain Mallory's hyaline and canalicular bile. It should be noted that, as in the case of liver cell adenomas, fatty change and Mallory's hyaline may be seen even in patients who do not drink.

Those nodules with atypical changes are termed 'dysplastic nodules' or 'atypical macroregenerative nodules'. In addition to the cytological changes (either of large cell or of small cell dysplasia), they also show architectural abnormalities. These architectural abnormalities may take the form of:

• a less cohesive growth pattern;
• focal loss of reticulin fibres; or
• the formation of pseudoaccini.

The presence of broad trabeculae should suggest the possibility of malignant change. Immunohistochemical staining for AFP is negative.

Particularly worrying features that suggest a high likelihood of progression to liver cell cancer are:

• small cell change;
• clear cell change; and
• fatty change.

Immunohistochemical markers, molecular biological markers and other markers of cell proliferation, such as AgNORs, have been suggested as being useful in distinguishing benign from malignant lesions. They tend not to be useful in individual cases, especially clinically difficult cases.

Hepatocellular carcinoma
Macroscopic appearance

Small HCCs are less than 4 cm in diameter. These may also be single or multiple. Macroscopically they may closely resemble macroregenerative nodules although the presence of necrosis or haemorrhage makes carcinoma more likely. HCCs are associated with either hepatitis B or hepatitis C usually arise in cirrhotic livers.

Microscopic appearance

Histological examination is necessary for distinguishing macroregenerative nodules from liver cell cancers. Malignant change is diagnosed on the basis of cytological features, growth pattern and immunophenotype. Although the cells in liver cell cancers resemble normal hepatocytes, they show:

- marked nuclear atypia;
- an increased nuclear–cytoplasmic ratio;
- an increased mitotic rate; and
- abnormal mitotic figures.

The degree of differentiation may vary markedly from area to area. Fatty change, Mallory's hyaline and eosinophilic intracytoplasmic inclusions, including α_1-antitrypsin bodies (even in patients who do not have α-antitrypsin deficiency), may be seen. Giant cell and clear cell variants have been described. Nevertheless it can be almost impossible to distinguish a well-differentiated HCC from a macroregenerative nodule or small cell dysplasia (see page 130) on the basis

of cytological features alone. It should be noted that there is no value in trying to grade liver cell carcinomas on the basis of a liver biopsy because such grading carries little prognostic information.

The recognition of an abnormal growth pattern is therefore essential to making the diagnosis of carcinoma (Figs 9.3 and 9.4). These tumours have trabeculae that range from a few cells in thickness to more than 20 cells in thickness and that are separated by endothelium-lined spaces. A very characteristic feature is the presence of very little, if any, supporting connective tissue. A reticulin stain is very helpful in confirming this. However, as is so often the case in histopathology, in the most difficult tumours this feature cannot be relied on for making the diagnosis. Focal fibrosis may be seen in otherwise typical liver cell cancers in areas of necrosis; fibrolamellar carcinomas in which fibrosis is a clinical feature are not associated with viral hepatitis or cirrhosis.

Another clue that a hepatocyte lesion is malignant is that the endothelial cells lining the sinusoids are CD34-positive; normal endothelial cells lining the hepatic sinusoids are CD34-negative.

A number of other growth patterns may be seen, including:

Figure 9.3
A fragment of a liver cell cancer with large cells with hyperchromatic nuclei arranged in a trabecular pattern.

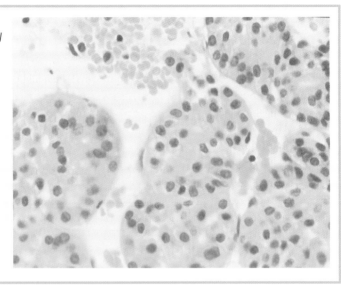

Figure 9.4
The same liver biopsy as in Figure 9.3, showing a marked decrease in reticulin staining compared with normal liver.

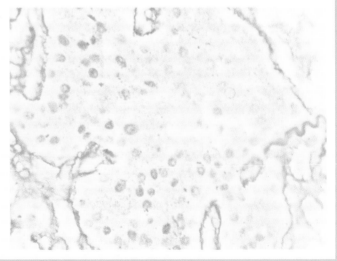

- a pseudoglandular pattern;
- a solid pattern; and
- a telangectatic pattern.

Capsular and vascular invasion, which is a very common feature in HCC, may be helpful in making the diagnosis. These variants need to be distinguished especially from metastatic carcinomas. Bile production, while uncommon, is diagnostic of liver cell carcinoma. HCC are frequently, albeit focally, positive for AFP. Although high serum AFP levels are common in HCC, positive immunohistochemical staining is much less commonly seen. Presumably this is because of the rapid rate at which this protein is secreted.

Similarly, staining for cytokeratins is sometimes useful in distinguishing liver cell carcinomas from other malignant tumours. If a tumour does not stain with AE1/AE3 (i.e. if it is negative for cytokeratins 7 and 20) then it is likely to be a HCC. On the other hand, if a tumour does not stain with AE1–AE3, this does not exclude the possibility that the tumour is a HCC since HCCs, like all other tumours, may show phenotypic differences from their non-neoplastic counterparts. A polyclonal antibody to carcinoembryonic antigen may be useful in identifying bile canaliculi in liver cell cancers.

Although HCC are overwhelmingly the most common malignancy seen in cirrhotic livers, cholangiocarcinomas and metastatic carcinomas should always be considered. It should be noted that adrenal cell carcinomas may also be positive for AFP. While the presence of coexisting cirrhosis makes it very likely that any tumour is a HCC, HCC can arise in non-cirrhotic livers. This is especially true in males living in areas where HCC is very common (e.g. Africa).

Management of the isolated hepatic nodule

Many patients with viral hepatitis develop a nodule within the liver. This is commonly identified during screening for hepatocellular carcinoma but similar lesions may be found during ultrasound examinations for other reasons (e.g. to investigate the upper abdominal pains that are common in patients with chronic hepatitis C). Accurate diagnosis is essential in this instance and the possible causes are listed in Table 9.2.

Most experienced ultrasonographers can identify cystic lesions and haemangiomas, and the clinician is left to decide the most

Table 9.2
Causes of an isolated liver nodule in patients with chronic viral hepatitis.

Lesion	Comments
Not related to viral liver disease	
Cystic lesions	Ususally simple hepatic cysts but cystadenomas and hydatid cysts should be considered
Haemangioma	Very common; can be diagnosed by MRI or contrast-enhanced CT scanning
Focal nodular hyperplasia	Rare; may require biopsy to confirm the diagnosis
Hepatic adenoma	Rare; tend to occur in women who have received oestrogens
Secondary tumour deposits	
Related to liver disease	
Regenerative nodules	Found in patients with cirrhosis, AFP may be raised
Primary liver cell cancer	

appropriate management of a solid hepatic nodule.

If the lesion is an HCC then a liver biopsy may spread the cancer along the needle tract and either on to the skin or throughout the peritoneal cavity. Tumour dissemination in this way causes significant morbidity and mortality and hence many hepatologists are reluctant to biopsy lesions that may be hepatocellular carcinoma. On the other hand, misdiagnosing a regenerative nodule as a liver cell cancer may have disastrous consequences. Although there is no consensus as to the most appropriate approach, we try to avoid liver biopsy in patients with proven cirrhosis who have large lesions (more than 4 cm in diameter) and who have a raised AFP level (over 500 ng/ml). Almost all of these lesions turn out to be HCC and biopsy provides little extra information. In other circumstances we find that a liver biopsy provides valuable diagnostic information; we perform an ultrasound-guided biopsy provided that there are no other contraindications.

During the biopsy it is important to take two samples of tissue – one sample should be taken from the lesion and one should be taken from the 'healthy tissue'. The importance of the second sample is that it allows the extent of the liver fibrosis to be determined – if there is coexisting cirrhosis (as is often the case) then resection of the lesion is not possible, but if there is minimal fibrosis then resection may be considered.

Management of hepatoceullar carcinoma

A full discussion of the management of liver cell cancer is beyond the scope of this volume, but a number of issues should be considered. In general, primary liver cell cancer is a very aggressive tumour that leads to death within a few months. However, a small proportion of patients have an indolent course and survive without therapy for many years. It is therefore essential that trials of novel therapeutic agents should be performed in large cohorts of patients with appropriate, untreated controls. The literature contains innumerable reports of 'effective' therapies for HCC that have been tested in small numbers of patients. Almost invariably, large, properly controlled studies demonstrate that these 'curative'

agents are of no value, and patients should be spared the side effects of chemotherapeutic regimens that have not been properly tested. At present there is no proven cytotoxic drug or combination of drugs that is beneficial, and patients with primary liver cell cancer should probably not receive chemotherapy outside the clinical trial setting.

Surgery for small HCCs that are found in non-cirrhotic livers may be curative, but careful patient selection is crucial; this approach should only be used by experienced surgeons who have low perioperative complication rates.

For patients with cirrhosis and HCC, early liver transplantation may be curative. However, the risk of recurrence in the new liver increases with the size of the original tumour, and most transplant centres will not operate on tumours that are greater than 4 cm in diameter. Tumour recurrence in the transplanted liver is always rapidly fatal. All patients with cirrhosis and early HCC should be discussed with the local transplant centre so that opportunities for transplantation are not missed.

For most patients with HCC and cirrhosis, the outlook is bleak. Local ablative therapy with either alcohol injection or thermoablation using laser fibres or cryoprobes have their advocates and may improve survival in some selected patients, but it is clear that experience in their use and careful selection of appropriate patients is necessary to achieve good results. It is therefore important that all patients with HCC are reviewed by clinicians with experience in the management of this disease so that those who may benefit from intervention are given the opportunity to benefit from the latest techniques.

Screening for HCC

It is clear that HCC can be cured only if it is detected at an early stage (when it is less than 4 cm in diameter). Since patients with cirrhosis caused by viral hepatitis are at high risk of developing HCC, many experts have advocated that these patients should be screened for early tumours by regular ultrasound examinations and serum AFP estimations. Many groups recommend an ultrasound every 6 months for all patients with cirrhosis and increase the frequency of screening to every 3 months in patients who are at high risk (i.e. those with an increased serum AFP level or dysplasia (see page 000).

Although this approach has much to

recommend it, it has not been subjected to any formal clinical trials, and its cost effectiveness has not been established. Our current policy is to discuss the merits of screening in patients who would be suitable for hepatic transplantation and to screen all those who agree to the procedure.

Dysplasia

Liver cell dysplasia has been shown to be associated with the development of HCC in patients with chronic hepatitis B. In seems likely that the same is true for patients infected with hepatitis C although this has not been proven. Most hepatologists agree that the presence of dysplasia on a liver biopsy increases the probability of HCC developing and accordingly they increase the intensity of monitoring or screening appropriately.

There are two forms of liver cell dysplasia:

- large cell dysplasia; and
- small cell dysplasia.

Liver cell dysplasia may been seen in macroregenerative nodules (see page 143) or on its own in either cirrhotic or non-cirrhotic livers. Clusters of large cell dysplasia or small cell dysplasia less than

1 mm in diameter have been termed 'dysplastic foci'. When they are seen in a macroregenerative nodules they are termed 'dysplastic nodules' (see page 143).

Large cell dysplasia

Large cell dysplasia is characterized by the presence of cells with large nuclei and increased amounts of cytoplasm (Fig. 9.5). This means that, despite the size of the nuclei, the nuclear–cytoplasmic ratio is normal. In addition to nuclear enlargement there may be pleomorphism and hyperchromasia as well as multinucleation and increased numbers of nucleoli. Recognition of this change is made easier if the size of normal hepatocytes, seen elsewhere in the biopsy, is used as an internal control.

Large cell dysplasia needs to be distinguished both from the increased nuclear pleomorphism seen in livers with increasing age and from the variability in nuclear size seen as a reactive change in livers with active lobular hepatitis. In addition to the presence of associated clinical and pathological features (i.e. patient's age, presence of active inflammation), another important clue is that the changes seen in liver cell dysplasia involve groups of contiguous

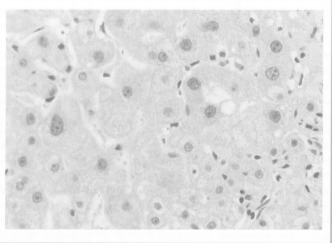

Figure 9.5
Liver biopsy from a patient with chronic hepatitis B. The cells in the top right of the picture contain sheets of hepatocytes with larger nuclei and more abundant cytoplasm. This is characteristic of large cell dysplasia. The nuclear–cytoplasmic ratio is normal.

hepatocytes rather than scattered cells. Image analysis is not necessary for diagnosing the presence of large cell dysplasia.

The nuclei in large cell dysplasia have been shown to be aneuploid and are associated with chromosomal abnormalities. Despite this, and although large cell dysplasia is associated with a four- to fivefold increased risk of coexisting HCC or of developing such a tumour, it is unlikely that the dysplastic cells are actually premalignant. Cell kinetic studies indicate that the proliferative rate of these cells is in fact

decreased. It has been suggested that large cell dysplasia may be the result either of a defect in 'polyploidization' or even chronic cholestasis.

Nevertheless the presence of large cell dysplasia, especially in patients with chronic hepatitis B, is taken as an indication that a patient needs careful follow-up with serum AFP and liver ultrasound.

Small cell dysplasia

In small cell dysplasia (Fig. 9.6), although the hyperchromatic nuclei are relatively

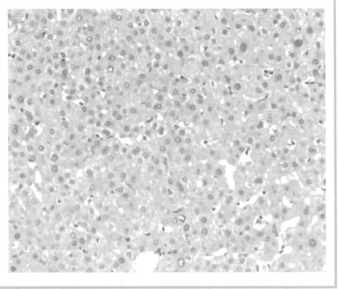

Figure 9.6
Liver biopsy showing nuclear crowding with cells with relatively small nuclei but with an increased nuclear–cytoplasmic ratio. This are the features of small cell dysplasia, which is more worrying than large cell dysplasia.

small and may actually be smaller than those seen in normal hepatocytes, because the cells themselves are smaller than usual, the nuclear cytoplasmic ration is increased. For unknown reasons, this change is considerably less common than large cell dysplasia in Western countries and Africa, whereas it is relatively common in Japan. When small cell dysplasia is seen it must be taken very seriously since it almost always means that there is coexistent HCC. The differential diagnosis from HCC can be very difficult.

Further reading

Arbuthnot P, Kew M. Hepatitis B virus and hepatocellular carcinoma. *Int J Exp Pathol* 2001; **82**: 77–100.

Colombo M. Hepatocellular carcinoma in patients with HCV. *Baillieres Clin Gastroenterol* 2000; **14**: 327–39.

Questions

1. Hepatocellular carcinoma:
   A. Is a very rare tumour
   B. May develop in patients with viral hepatitis who do not have cirrhosis
   C. May be cured by transplantation
   D. Is radiosensitive
   E. The diagnosis needs to be confirmed by liver biopsy

2. An isolated hepatic nodule:
   A. If found in a patient with cirrhosis caused by viral hepatitis is always malignant
   B. May be due to a regenerative nodule
   C. Should be investigated by performing a serum AFP estimation
   D. Must be benign if the serum AFP level is normal
   E. Should be imaged using angiography to exclude haemangioma

3. Histological features of a hepatocellular carcinoma include:
   A. Preservation of liver architecture
   B. Little, if any, connective tissue
   C. Nuclear atypia
   D. Bile production
   E. Absence of fatty change, which excludes the diagnosis

4. Regarding cirrhosis due to viral hepatitis:
   A. Dysplasia is associated with an increased risk of developing HCC
   B. Secondary tumours are commoner than primary tumours
   C. Only patients with cirrhosis are at risk of developing HCC

D. There is an increased risk of developing fibrolamellar HCC
E. It never leads to cancer if the patient has received interferon therapy

Answers

Question 1

A. False – world-wide, primary hepatocellular carcinoma is the most common malignant tumour
B. True
C. True
D. False
E. False

Question 2

A. False – regenerative nodules are common in this setting
B. True
C. True
D. False – 50% of HCCs have a normal serum AFP
E. False

Question 3

A. False
B. True
C. True
D. True
E. False

Question 4

A. True
B. False
C. False
D. False
E. False

Index

55–65
associated liver autoantibodies 63–4
children 64–5
drug users, active 62–3
management during therapy 61–2
pretreatment assessment 59–61
computed tomography scanning 138, 140, 141
concentration, difficulty in 52, 116
confluent necrosis 39
connective tissue 145
consensus interferon 55
contraceptive precautions 59
contrast administration 140–1
core proteins 3, 21, 73
corticosteroids 121
cough 54, 63
covalently closed, circular DNA (cccDNA) 70
cryocrit 117, 118
cryoglobulinaemia 117, 118, 120
cryoglobulins 117, 120
cryoprobes 150
cyclophosphamide 121
cytokines 2, 6, 8n, 55
cytological features 145
cytomegalovirus 86
cytopathic liver cell damage 81
cytoplasm 151
     granular 78
cytoplasmic staining 81, 106
cytoplasmic vacuolation 29
cytosine 104
cytotoxic agents 86, 141
cytotoxic CD8–positive T lymphocytes 81

decompensation 99
defective proteins 70
delta antigens 104, 106
delta virus 1, 15–16, 81, 103–9
     antigens 106
     diagnosis 105–6
     management 107–9
     natural history 104–5
     pathology 106–7
     replication 104

superinfection 91
dendritic cells 26
dengue virus 20
depression 61, 63, 96, 98, 116
dermatitis, acropapular 122
dialysis 132
difficult-to-treat patient groups 125–35
     cirrhosis 125–31
     immunosuppressive medication 131–3
DNA 109, 133
     covalently closed circular 70
drug abuse *see* intravenous drug use
dyplastic nodules 143–4
dysplasia 81, 83, 84, 150–3
dysplastic foci 151
dysplastic nodules 142–3, 144, 151

E1 protein 21
E2 portal 3
Egypt 10, 33
electrocardiogram 59
electron microscopy 122
endocrinology 120
endoplasmic reticulum 23, 73
endoscopy 126
endothelial cells 145
endothelium-lined spaces 145
envelope protein 21, 23, 70, 95, 104
enzyme immunoassay 47–8
enzyme-inducing drugs 78
epitopes 8
Epstein-Barr virus 30
erythropoetin 54
ethnic groups 13, 121
Europe 9, 10, 13, 52

family history 119
family members, infection from 12
Far East 13, 22
Fas/Fasl interactions 6
fatigue 52, 54, 116, 119
fatty change 26, 29, 106, 144, 145
fever 61, 120
fibrinogen storage disease 78

position 1015 104
precore mutant B virus 76
precore region 76
precore-core 73
prednisolone 63, 64
pregnancy screening 59
prevalence 9–16
 B virus 13–15
 C virus 9–12
 delta virus 15–16
proinflammatory cytokines 2
promiscuity 11, 12, 14, 16
prophylaxis, primary 126
propranolol 126
protease inhibitors 23
protein:
 CD81 22
 core 3, 21, 73
 defective 70
 E1 21
 envelope 21, 23, 70, 95, 104
 helicase 23
 ISG 15 4
 ISG 54 4
 kinase (PKR) 2–3, 4
 lytic 6
 Mx 3, 4
 non-structural 23
 NS2–4 23
 NS5 3, 23
 POL 70, 73
 polymerase 3, 23, 70, 98
 structural 73
 surface 70, 72–3
 TAP 6
 tetraspanin 22
 YMDD 98
proteosome 6
prothrombin index 77, 99
pseudoaccini 144
psychiatric disorders 52, 61, 98, 115, 116
psychoses 63
pulmonary disease 59
pyoderma gangrenosum 120

quasispecies 20

receptors:
 cell surface 21
 IL-12 3, 4
 TOLL-like family of 2
recombinant modified interferon 55
recombinant naturally occurring interferons 55
regenerative liver nodules 138
resting pulse rate 126
reticulin fibres 144
reticulin stain 26, 145
retroviruses 70
reverse transcriptase 73
 inhibitors 95, 100, 1311
rheumatoid arthritis 131
rheumatoid factor 117
RIBA assays 47–8
ribavirin:
 B virus and C virus co-infection 110
 C virus 22, 33, 42, 53, 54–5
 cirrhosis 126, 127
 HIV and C virus co-infection 111
 immunohistochemical staining 52
 immunosuppressive medication 132
 non-hepatic manifestations and C virus 118
 see also combination therapy
ribosomes 22
ribozyme 104
RNA 20, 23, 48, 109, 117
 antigenomic 104
 genome 104
 intermediate 70
 pregenomic 70
 replicating 2
RNase 73
rolling circle mechanism 104
Romania 16

sanded nuclei 106
sarcoidosis 30
Sardinia 10
Scandinavia 9
scarring 24